POSITIVELY
WOMEN

LIVING WITH AIDS

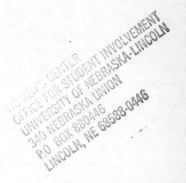

POSITIVELY WOMEN

LIVING WITH AIDS

EDITED BY
SUE O'SULLIVAN
& KATE THOMSON

SHEBA
FEMINIST
PRESS

First published in Britian in 1992 by Sheba Feminist Press,
10A Bradbury Street, London N16 8JN.

Cover illustration by Pam Skelton, detail from 'In the Land of Culture'
Cover and inside design by Spark Ceresa
Typeset by Photosetting and Secretarial Services, Yeovil, England
Printed and bound by Cox & Wyman Ltd, Reading, England

British Library Cataloguing in Publication Data
A record for this book is available from the British Library

ACKNOWLEDGEMENTS

Among the many people who have given inspiration, help and guidance during the creation of this book special thanks go to friends and family, in particular: Sona, Allison, Joan, Sarah, Paul, Janey and John. Grateful thanks to Sheba for being patient and excited; the Women's Solidarity Fund for much needed financial help; Rita O'Brien; Ellen Mizzel, Sue Katz and Prue Cave for transcribing the first tapes; friends of Sheba in particular Pip Salvador-Jones and RaeAnn Robertson; Positively Women staff for time and energy; every single woman who came to the Spring Cruise event in April 1991 and helped both Sheba and Positively Women continue their work; Sara Dunn for editorial advice; Mitch Cleary for computer loans and help; and most of all to each woman who generously agreed to be part of this book.

Sue O'Sullivan: During the creation of this book I have made wonderful friends, especially Kate Thomson, Fiona and Sheila. Mitch has supported me emotionally and practically all along and only she will know how much this meant to me. I have valued the talks about HIV and AIDS with my two sons, Tom and Dan. Thanks too, to all of my friends and to Jean Smith in particular, who came through for me with bells on, even when she grumbled.

Kate Thomson: Love and thanks to my family; to all the members and staff at Positively Women; to Peter Nevins, Peter Griffith, Geoff, Hamad, Kevin and Sean; to Sue O'Sullivan, Sue Papa, Sheila, Mathew, Fiona, Caroline and Yanne; and most of all to my sister, Rachel. Without your patience and support this book would not have been possible.

FOR LORI

To every single person,
no matter what their HIV status,
who stands up for people
living with HIV and AIDS,
and to every organization
fighting for our lives.

CONTENTS

INTRODUCTION

THIS IS A book by positive women about their lives and their hopes, as well as the problems they have faced. Women who work in the HIV and AIDS field have also contributed pieces which offer information and develop issues of importance to understanding the specific hurdles which positive women face. It is not necessarily a book to be read from cover to cover. It can be savoured a bit at a time, contemplated and picked up again.

The beginnings of the book go way back. In early 1987 Positively Women was an idea in one positive woman's mind. Soon afterwards an unassuming flyer appeared which announced the setting up of a self-help group for positive women. Slowly but surely women responded and the organization grew. The editors of this book met while doing publicity for the new organization and after long and fruitful talks the possibility of a book which would tell the stories of positive women in their own words took shape.

The book making process began - one which ended up taking years to finish. At the start, we decided to edit the book ourselves. Sue was the Sheba editor and Kate and another woman were the Positively Women editors. During the process of creating the book, the third woman had to withdraw from that role.

From the beginning all three of us were determined that positive women should be able to tell their own stories; initially we thought most of the women would want to write these themselves. In fact, the task of writing alone, and in most cases for the first time, was daunting and finally the majority of the women chose to be interviewed by either Kate or Sue and then to work from the transcript. This process is a lengthy one - in some cases so much time elapsed after an interview that we had the chance to go back to the same woman and get an update. The long delays have been frustrating but on the other hand doing two separated interviews illustrated the fluidity of women's attitudes and circumstances. Women who are positive are no less subject to changes in their lives and feelings about being HIV positive than anyone else is about the circumstances of their lives.

We also decided that although this book is not primarily a 'handbook' for HIV positive women, it would be crazy to miss the opportunity to put in information and ideas about HIV from people working in the field - either as health practitioners, service providers or activists. So we have interviewed doctors, alternative health practitioners, an AIDS and housing worker, a legal worker, a midwife, a drugs worker, and Positively Women staff workers. We have also provided a currently up-to-date resource guide.

We see this book as having a number of roles. Most importantly, it is a book which will be read by other positive women who may still be experiencing total isolation and silence. Over and over again the women in this book tell of their own feelings of being alone in their positive status, of the necessity for keeping it completely secret or of having to choose very, very carefully the people they could tell. By courageously opening up their lives these women are cutting through the invisibility which still surrounds the majority of women living with HIV.

We have asked women to go beyond their HIV experiences and to tell us about their lives, their histories, their relationships, in order to contextualize their HIV status. Positive women are NOT just sad victims or famous people: they are wonderfully ordinary; they are diverse; they are a hundred other things besides being HIV positive; they are all living with HIV; they could be anyone - you or your neighbour or your sister or your lover.

Of course the complexities and influences of different cultures, class inequalities, immigration status, race, age, and sexuality implode on the HIV positive woman. The truth of the matter is that as women are second-class citizens in society, so too are they second-class participants in the AIDS crisis. In the USA it has been noted that women living with AIDS die sooner than their white, gay, male counterparts. Why should this be? We can only surmise that a significant aspect of it will have to do with the fact that women tend to be poorer, to be diagnosed later because specifically female conditions which might indicate the presence of HIV are still not officially recognized as HIV related, such as thrush or pre-cancerous cervical changes, and because women's health is often of less concern than men's.

The women's stories make clear the bonding which takes place between them because of the virus. Their experiences also help to clarify the need to break down any notion of a 'universal' approach to HIV and AIDS and to illustrate that language about sexuality, relationships, health, and work can not assume that women are all the same.

So this book is about the empowerment which can come through sharing and claiming a common experience, *and* about the differences between women. But it is also about telling others that 'we are here'. Listen to us, look at us, see yourselves in us. One of the most destructive aspects of AIDS is the stigma and fear which loads it down. For many people, HIV and AIDS implies so much more than the condition itself. Too much blaming goes on. In a society which is racist and anti-gay, and exhibits a heavy dose of drugs hysteria, people who are HIV positive often get blamed because of who they are, or because they have had the misfortune to make love without protection with someone who is HIV positive, or have shared dirty needles.

Now, with the numbers of women who are contracting the virus through heterosexual sex rising, the imaginary and dangerously false division between 'them' and 'us' is breaking down. In this book we would like to demystify and make ordinary ALL women's experiences of becoming HIV positive. The stigma and fear around HIV must be broken down. On its own, it does great harm to those who are positive, who must bear the burden of the fear and stigma at the same time that they are attempting to deal with their own hopes and fears. And it does harm to the people who stigmatize and fear, compromising their humanity and making them into perpetrators of violence and ostracism, even if they don't directly carry out any deeds.

As is so often the case in a book which is a 'first', we have not been able to include everything we wanted to. Some contributions fell through at the last minute, others we were unable to cover ourselves. The most obvious examples are prostitution and intravenous drug use. Many women in the book talk about their intravenous drug involvement, but no one addresses the reality of prostitution. However, we have included useful material in the RESOURCES section.

Sex workers have been stigmatized as transmitters of HIV, 'bad' women who are a danger to their clients (and their clients' families). In fact, the majority of sex workers are more conscious of the importance of safer sex practice than other people having sex with men. It is the sex worker who is at the blunt end of the legal system, society's condemnation, poverty and violence from clients and pimps and who is in most danger of HIV infection *from* her clients, who may insist on unprotected sex. A sex worker who also uses drugs intravenously is more probably at risk from HIV through sharing dirty needles than through selling sex. It is always important to remember that the issue is 'high risk behaviour', not 'high risk groups'. No one, including sex workers, must be scapegoated for HIV transmission.

Many heterosexually-identified men find it 'easier' to blame a prostitute for their HIV status, rather than admitting to sex with other men, or intravenous drug use. Many women find it difficult to talk openly about being a sex worker. Despite being the 'oldest profession', sex work is still one of the strictest taboos throughout the world.

We hope that anyone, indeed everyone, will be able to read this book and identify with some part of it, so that the separation between those who are positive and those who assume they are not will be made smaller, and the stigma of the virus lessened.

Positively Women is the first autonomous women's HIV/AIDS organization to exist in this country. However, it's important to recognize that it forms part of a constellation of voluntary sector responses to the AIDS crisis. Groups such as the Terrence Higgins Trust, Landmark, the Lighthouse, and many local support groups and help lines, continue to have an important role in providing services, support, and education to men and women affected by HIV. These groups, to varying degrees have responded to the needs of women. What makes Positively Women unique and necessary is its undivided focus on the needs of women. What the woman who started Positively Woman identified as her own needs as a positive woman - to address the specificity of being a woman and being positive - remain the touchstone of the organization.

Positively Woman is there for any woman who is positive. The largest number of women in the organization at the beginning were ex or current drug users, but this has changed significantly in the past few years. Now as many women who have contracted the virus through heterosexual sex are taking part in Positively Women. Also the numbers of African women based in Britain and lesbians have grown. Positively Women is the women who come to it - its policy is open rather than exclusive. Of course questions of race, class and sexuality are not that easily overcome and accesibility of the organization to different groups of women is sometimes problematic. But the staff who run Positively Women (some positive and some not), and the women who use its services and support groups are committed to finding ways to keep it open and at the same time to recognize that all women do not have the same needs. Positively Women is an organization in process - it is not static or unchangeable. One obvious problem is that the organization is London-based; clearly there is a need for similar groups in other areas of Britain. Positively Women is keen to help groups set up in other cities.

Women who are positive want and need many different things from the organization. Perhaps the most obvious are services and support groups. These are being carefully considered, at the same time that already existing work is consolidated. Another important side of work is advocacy and education through speaking to a wide variety of groups, as well as pressuring and working with appropriate governmental and intergovernmental bodies such as the World Health Organization (WHO), for more recognition of women's needs, research, funding, service support, input into policy making, and for human rights.

Positively Women also attempts to make international links. In a world context, AIDS primarily affects heterosexuals and within that category women are affected greatly. Not only can information be shared, solidarity too can be expressed across national boundaries.

The women at Positively Women are mainly heterosexual although there is growing recognition that there are HIV positive lesbians, usually through needle use or the occasional sexual encounter with men. Many HIV/AIDS organizations in this country were started by the first group of people affected by the virus, gay men. The work they have done to organize their communities and to reach out to others has been admirable. And yet, their experience as gay men has often meant that their understanding of women's issues and experiences has had limitations. Positively Women has seen a need for a group which validates women's experiences, without being separatist in any way. The organization maintains open and helpful links with other HIV/AIDS organizations and with the people, many of them gay, who work with such dedication. In the same way that Positively Women wants to make and keep international links with groups of HIV positive women, it wants to keep links with other groups in this country working on the same issues - be they mixed, black, gay, drug oriented, or aimed at sex workers. It does this from an autonomous position of strength, willing to learn and to inform.

There is no clear 'line' in this book about what is appropriate treatment for people who have any of the illnesses associated with either an HIV status or with AIDS. We have included information and experiences which indicate a range of possible choices. At this time there is no absolute certainty about any form of medical or alternative treatment in relation to those illnesses. Some women will choose to follow their doctor's advice and go on AZT or other allopathic drug treatments, others will chose acupuncture, herbs, homeopathy, diet or meditation, while others (the majority in this book) will try to combine Western treatment with alternative approaches. Again and again women reiterate that choice, information, and flexibility is most important to them. Feeling good about what health measures you follow seems to make people actually feel better physically and mentally.

We would also like to make it crystal clear that whatever form of treatment a woman living with HIV follows, it is not her fault if a particular approach doesn't work for her. Many people are quite rightly critical of the drug oriented treatments of Western medicine, but we are also critical of any suggestion that if you are a 'good enough' person, or follow an holistic approach 'well enough' you will get better, and if you don't get better the fault lies with you. This is rubbish.

The majority of positive women in the book have had to remain anonymous. We have decided to use first names only in all of their stories in order to underline the difficulty they face in 'coming out'. Telling their stories in the first place was a brave act. The necessity to remain anonymous is an indication of the very real oppression which HIV positive people face from society - from other people and from officialdom - if they go public. It's a vicious circle: until women (and men) can more easily be open about their status, they will remain hidden and 'other'. But until they can be out without undue fear of reprisals and ostracism, they aren't able to do so. Here women speak out. We must all take part in making it a society in which they can do so under their own names. The few women who are public must eventually be joined by others. We hope this book helps to change feelings and opinions and makes that a little more possible.

Kate Thomson and Sue O'Sullivan
London, March 1992

POSITIVELY WOMEN: STATEMENT OF AIMS AND SERVICES

POSITIVELY WOMEN started as a small self-help group in 1987. It has grown into the major national organization for women with HIV and AIDS in Britain with its headquarters in London.

The organization's main aims are:

1. To protect the health of women, particularly by provision of counselling and support services to women who are living with HIV and AIDS or any associated condition.
2. To advance education and research about women's health and particularly the health of those who are living with HIV and AIDS or any associated condition.
3. To provide community centred advice and assistance and undertake any other charitable activity for the benefit of women living with HIV and AIDS or any associated condition.

Peer support is the key to the organization's services and is available through a range of options, including support groups, one-to-one and telephone counselling sessions, hospital and home visits, open days and social events.

For full details, including address, telephone numbers and services provided, please see Resources, page 295.

POSITIVE WOMEN

OUR LIVES, OUR STORIES

SHEILA

Sheila is thirty-six, has been positive for eight years and has had AIDS for the last three. She has been through much, but has survived.

REBELLIOUSNESS WAS BORN in me. I had a sister who was very good academically; never put a foot wrong, went to teachers training college, had nice, middle-class friends. But my mum had been on the stage before she had us and because I was creative, she put a lot of energy into me. I was the little performer. Alice got the positive attention, and I went for the negative. When I was younger I could get away with it because it was funny; I'd be the cheeky one who made the grown-ups laugh. I would think nothing of getting up and singing a song and dancing in front of everyone. My mum loved it and she had expectations that I would go into the theatre or be a rock star.

The older I got, the less funny it all was and I became quite bitter. I'd see Alice still doing everything perfectly. It started going wrong at about twelve or thirteen when I began smoking dope, taking pills and drinking. With hindsight I can see I was rebelling against my parents' Scottish middle-classness. Out of all the girls in my class at school, I was the only one whose parents had bought their house and I hated it. We used to speak really posh when we were younger, but as I grew up I quickly acquired a Glaswegian accent. I made my parents miserable; they didn't know what to do with me. I was a real problem, a troublesome 1970s teenager - police files, shop-lifting, bunking off school, you name it. The group of girls I hung around with were called Townies because we came from Glasgow. We thought we had real style - tight straight jeans with suit jackets. The shop-lifting wasn't necessarily done to get money for drugs. I shop-lifted partly for the sake of doing it and partly for drugs money. I'd go into Boots and steal a make-up bag, fill it with things for myself or to take into school to sell.

I've always had a lot of energy and I couldn't find a positive outlet for it. If I hadn't ended up on heroin it's likely I might have settled with someone and had children, but that's guess work.

I lost my virginity when I was sixteen which was relatively old when you think about it. Where I come from you got slagged off, called a cow, a dirty whore, if you lost your virginity, so it was a big thing when it happened. I lost it to my first real boy-friend Gary and the second time I slept with him I got pregnant, a fact I didn't realize until I was three or four months gone and even then it was my mum who figured it out.

The decision about what to do was taken out of my hands and my parents brought in a doctor friend of theirs. I was five months pregnant when I had the abortion. It was a terrible experience but it wasn't until much later that I recognized the damage it had done to me. When the baby came away, a horrible stern-faced witch of a nurse cut it away, and put it in tissue paper - all in full view. After that trauma I left home - I was sixteen years old. My dad has since asked me if I think the abortion had anything to do with the way the rest of my life unfolded. I think he's felt a lot of guilt about taking that decision. I might have had the baby if left on my own, but I also think I was relieved when the decision was made for me.

I came to England and ended up in London where I started off doing secretarial work and got a little flat in Tufnell Park along with some other people. I led a relatively straight life for about two years. I always smoked dope and took a bit of speed but that was all; then it got to be quite a lot of speed, and finally it got to be everyday. I can't remember much about those first two years, but I guess it was pretty boring. We went to rock concerts and parties; in a way it was all quite innocent with no real heaviness except for the amount of speed we took.

I went to work in a children's home as a house parent for the youngest kids, but I left, with some of the other staff, after we protested about the Victorian punishments the head of the home handed out to the children; I could never keep my mouth shut!

During the first few years in London heroin wasn't in the picture. However, I had developed a big needle fixation through injecting speed a few times; there was something about putting a needle in my arm I loved, perhaps the fascination was about having total power and control as you're the only one involved. Even now at the hospital I take my own blood because I can't handle anybody else putting a needle into me.

By then I'd moved to a Hackney squat in a long street of other squatted houses across from Victoria Park which was absolutely fantastic. Some wonderful people lived on that street and I ended up living there off and on for quite a few years. I had no real direction in my life except that I was starting to dabble in drugs more heavily. I travelled - to Kent for hop picking, over to Morocco for a few months, then to Spain.

Back in Hackney, with my budding career in the children's home over, I lived on the dole. Our house was open - everyone coming from Scotland came to stay with us at first. We were noisy and riotous; we got drunk and stoned, and we had a wonderful time. The whole street was one big open house, nothing was locked up, and the atmosphere was great.

After travelling some more, I returned to Hackney and found everything changing. Serious heroin users had arrived on the scene and quite a few of us started using too. The character of the street altered, people started closing their doors to stop things getting nicked, the trust we'd shared was gone.

Around this time I went on a trip to Italy and met an Australian journalist living in Rome who suggested I train with him. It was all really enjoyable and exciting. I had dinner with Richard Burton and Suzy Hunt, met John Travolta and all his family. I'd take our stories back to London to sell on Fleet Street!

I met Mario during a trip back to England, fell madly in love with him, gave up trying to be a journalist immediately, and moved back to England. Mario was an Italian who'd come here to get rid of a heroin habit - which he didn't get rid of.

For me, it all started here, the serious heroin use. He and I were a using couple for ten years; we depended on each other completely. I was totally in love with him, sexually besotted. People think heroin ruins your sex life but it never happened to us. Eventually he got deported and we spent four years together in Italy. Although I loved him, he beat the shit out of me. For nine years not a day passed when I didn't have a bruise on me. I hated it but I loved him and our mutual dependence made it impossible for me to extricate myself. I still hurt a lot when I think what I let myself go through in that relationship. I tried to leave him many times but I could never get rid of him. He would come after me, I would capitulate, and we would go back to Italy again. Once I managed to leave for eighteen months to stay with my family in Scotland while I tried to get off drugs completely. But I ended up hitting the drink which was worse than drugs. It may sound strange but given the choice I preferred being a drug addict to an alcoholic. Finally after ten years we separated. I'm not in touch with Mario now so I have no idea what's happening to him except that he too is HIV.

I took heroin for the first time when I was living in Spain for a few months. It was a glamorous, romantic situation and I loved everything about taking it. I thought: right, when I go back to London, this is what I am going to do. And for about ten years I did what I set out to do and became a dealer. When I was with Mario in Italy we had Mafia connections and made thousands and thousands of pounds. It was dangerous at times; once we owed about £100 to the boss and although we had the money to pay him, because we were addicts and chaotic, we took the money and scored instead. That night we were walking home when two guys stepped out of a doorway, put a bread knife right into Mario and turned it. He nearly died. Later, when we started getting into coke and the money was going down, my ankle was smashed by someone trying to extract money from me. They wouldn't knock you off, but they would do things like that to serve as a warning: of course we'd tell other street dealers what happened to us which broadcast the message and made the point.

I never sold to kids. We sold specifically to people who came to the parks to buy; if they didn't buy off of us, it would have been someone else. I've bloody bought off some people for years, so I've no guilt about selling to others. Maybe some anger about non-users who sell. I think there should be two laws: one for the guys who don't use and sell who are exploiting addicts; and one for the users who only sell to keep their own habit. Most of the time it's pathetic; someone buys half a gram of heroin and then makes up three bags to get money back to buy another half gram, and then they'll be able to have a fix. These people are labelled as dealers but they're not really and they get the same sentences as the guys who don't use but make large amounts of money out of it. Dealers like us never made money because we spent it all on our habit. We put thousands of pounds up our arms.

For a couple of years after I was diagnosed HIV positive, I wandered about pretty aimlessly, trying to stay off drugs without much success. I couldn't cope alone. It was early days in relation to AIDS, when people were frightened and ignorant, and as a result I suffered a lot of rejection. So I went back to using, to the people I knew who accepted me for who I was. They didn't really have enough caring in them to worry if I had the virus or not, it was neither here nor there to them, which suited me fine.

But they certainly cared more than what I experienced when reading what the media had to say about people with AIDS, and more than existed in the drug rehabilitation units and street agencies I came in contact with.

At one drug rehab unit I was told to leave because I tried to talk about being positive - they didn't want to know. I know

now how much that affected me, but at the time I was in such a mess I didn't realize the hurt it caused. At another I stole money, took a taxi back into London, and went straight out and scored. That's what the place did for me. But I kept trying; I went to Narcotics Anonymous and in a meeting, when I tried to 'share' my experience of being positive a couple of people got up and walked out. I was devastated. I could make excuses for rejection from recovering alcoholics and straight staff, but I couldn't for the people in Narcotics Anonymous because I thought of them as my 'own' people. I gave up again and went back to using but in the back of my mind I knew if I carried on my body was going to conk out and I would kill myself.

I'm in my thirties now. At one time I loved duckin' and divin' about on the streets, but I wouldn't now; I'm too old for it. For years I was a dealer with a lot of status, a lot of junkie respect. Giving it all up, you go from being the queen of a little crowd to being a nobody in the big wide world. It's part of my personality to try to get things done, to organize things in any situation I find myself in. My mum used to say she always knew I would succeed in something, but she never dreamt it would be in the AIDS field. In fact I succeeded in being a heroin addict. My decision was clear-cut: I wanted to be one. Even when my body was a wreck I didn't see it that way. You look at the mirror through heroin eyes. Through those eyes my gaunt face looked lovely, although I hate the look now. I thought I looked great because I was absolutely out of my head. The only thing that bothered me towards the end (and it bothers me now) was my track marks. But at that point I was in such a rebellious state I would roll up my sleeves in order to show them to the world.

Before trying to give up, I ended up in hospital with pneumonia, pleurisy, septicemia, and growths on my lungs and on the valve which pumps blood in through the heart. Believe me, I had hit rock-bottom with a thump. After being discharged I didn't take enough time for physical or mental recovery before I went back on drugs and I could literally feel my body going downhill again. I knew I had to try to clean up again so I went to the City Roads rehab centre. I was their first identified HIV positive client and in many ways I was a great experience for them because a lot of people got their AIDS learning through me. Because I understood perfectly well what was happening I was happy to take on that role. It gave me a measure of self-worth because I was teaching them at the same time as being their 'client'.

I could never ever class myself as a drug user who really needed help, although I see now that I had a problem. I always felt I was more sussed out and different from other people. I often turned the street agencies I used around and was helpful to them and they recognized it. When I was at Phoenix House everyone was fine about my HIV status except I could never get away from the virus. One-to-one counselling or heavy confrontational groups were part of our programme but I was never allowed to have other problems without someone saying, 'Never mind about that. What about the virus? You're avoiding it, you're in denial.' Couldn't they understand that, yes, it was a big problem - but so was my drug using, so were the problems I had around relationships. It was as if they were denying me the right to talk about anything else. Ironically being HIV positive gave me a lot of status even though it was a distorted kind of status. When you're in places like that, you tend to play games. That's all very well - I could give and take, play around with the drama a bit, but I always knew what I was doing.

All along and underneath, my deep down needs were not being met which was very depressing. I had nobody to tell about all my feelings who could turn around and say, 'God, I know how you feel, I've been through it too.' I went to a few HIV/AIDS support groups which were very gay-orientated which was fine, because they were doing a great job supporting each other, but it wasn't fine for me because my needs weren't being met. I was always the only woman and when I turned up knew the conversations would be very different. Some of the men quite subtly and nicely told me it was a refreshing change because they talked about different issues when I was there. I was isolated; they thought of me as being so different that it didn't really matter where I was from, or what I had done.

I was out of Phoenix House into what they term the re-entry part of the programme, where you live in a shared house while you wait for your own flat. I turned thirty and had a lot more freedom and time and I was still waiting around for something to be done for HIV positive women and nothing was happening. Then one day I just thought: okay, if no one else is going to do it, I will. It was as simple as that. I sat down and wrote: 'If you are a woman who has HIV or AIDS and would like to talk to another woman who has the same, then please ring this number.' I went to Women's Reproductive Rights Information Centre and they let me use the photocopier and gave me the stamps, as well as a huge list of addresses of all the women's centres, hospitals and drug rehabs - everywhere a woman might come into contact with my amateur poster. Phoenix gave me the paper. SCODA (Standing Committee on Drugs and Alcohol) gave me a room to use once a fortnight.

Slowly but surely the phone calls came in and a support group started. I got my flat and started spending more time working on the group. Everything got a bit more organized, we got a proper poster, the group was going well, and many more women started turning up. Those other women made such a difference to my life. I wasn't the only woman in Britain who had this bloody virus, because I'll tell you, I really felt like that before.

Meanwhile, I was going to the hospital where HIV positive women were a new phenomenon. All the students and doctors wanted to meet and talk to us; they were probing us for information. It's unbelievable what guinea pigs we were. I handled it well because I was now organizing and getting support and had a lot invested in making Positively Women a success. I had reclaimed some self-esteem: I wasn't just a piece of shit, a parasitical ex-drug user who had the virus. Maybe there were still people who would put me down, but that started to be immaterial. What mattered was that I was in touch with women from all walks of life who were getting something from the group, and through that I did too. Positively Women's reputation grew and I started giving talks to other organizations on the personal aspects of having HIV. I was on the way to being well known within the AIDS field by health authorities, local councils, hospitals, as well as other AIDS organizations. I even started getting a business head and charged a speaker's fee! After giving free talks for two years, I thought, everyone else is getting paid, maybe I should. Positively Women progressed and progressed - sadly out of necessity because the numbers of HIV positive women grew and we had to deal with that. We're still dealing with a minority of the women who are affected by AIDS and HIV in this country but we've managed to make a big impact nevertheless.

We've been lucky at Positively Women to learn from other peoples' mistakes. We've also kept our services to a basic minimum and are aware that it's necessary to build and strengthen them before we take on anything else. The first women at the core of Positively Women, the skills that Kate, Fiona, Pearl and I had were very complementary. Personally, I don't like co-operatives, I had experience of them in the past and I never found they worked very well. At Positively Women we have conformed to a hierarchical structure for funding reasons primarily, but I believe that leaders can be valuable to organizations. All the workers should have choices and input at work, but I think it works best when someone has the responsibility to make final decisions.

I believe that power should stay primarily with positive people in any organization working on their behalf. On a larger scale my argument is that there are an awful lot of people making decisions for people living with HIV and AIDS, and they don't fully understand the situation. That's why it's so important that people like me have a say over what happens. After all, it's our lives we're talking about.

I have a big investment in my role as a facilitator and carer and I understand that it gives me power and status. But I'm aware of not looking after myself enough and not taking enough care of my own mental and physical needs. I've been under far too much strain for a long time and I'm completely burned out. This knowledge is intertwined with other feelings about Positively Women. I see Positively Women as 'my baby', a baby I never fully want to let it go of. I find it difficult to trust other women 100 per cent to run it without me being in final control. It took me a while to come to terms with the fact that the organization could run without me. It's a strange contradiction because the realization was both hurtful and a relief. For instance, when I was in hospital and a Positively Women decision was made without consulting me, I was angry - how dare decisions about Positively Women be made without conferring with me? I also felt jealousy and resentment when other women got recognition for their work. Where did all these emotions came from and how could I deal with them? I've resolved many of these conflicts although I'd be lying if I said they were completely gone. I am recognized for playing a central role in bringing the issue of HIV and women to the fore and for highlighting things other women might not have thought about.

We've had heated discussions at Positively Women about how those of us who run the organization and are HIV positive or have AIDS can get our needs met. At one point I was told I shouldn't be using the group when I was in a bad way because the other women had me up on a pedestal, and thought of me as eternally happy, strong and positive thinking; to see my weaknesses would scare them. This came up around the time I had been dabbling with drugs a little and I wanted to talk about it in a group. When I was advised not to, I reminded them that I set up the organization because I wasn't getting support anywhere else. It was a ironic to be told now that I shouldn't be using Positively Women for my problems because of other HIV postive women.

I believe that letting other women think we're continuously

strong and positive is wrong and would be doing them no favours. In reality we're human, we can't be perfect all the time. The women coming to Positively Women now have to know that those of us who set the organization up are imperfect and that we have contradictions in our own lives. Otherwise when they go through bad times it will be worse; they'll think, how come I can't do it perfectly if they can? That could make them feel like failures.

I live for the day. What happens is meant to happen. Instead of feeling angry straight away, I now try to analyse difficult situations and see what positive things can come out of them. I don't want to be misunderstood. I am not thankful I have AIDS because it has made me a 'better person'. The idea that you can become a better person through having the virus makes me angry. I've become more aware of a lot of things since I was diagnosed, but what a fucking hell of a way to go about it! It makes me sad that it had to take something like this for me to arrive where I am today. But I'm not all virus. AIDS has been a part of it, but that's not what I'm all about. My changes have to do as much with becoming a mother and my age. Given the choice of a perfect world, I would not want to be where I am today for the same reasons. I'll take it one step further. I've heard of people who wished they had the virus because they see something in a positive person they want in themselves and because they're frustrated with their own lives they focus on the virus. It's a poor thing, and a shame that it takes a crisis to bring out the best in people.

I've had times when I've gone back to what I know which is using heroin. It doesn't necessarily indicate that I'm depressed; it might be the opposite. Perhaps I believe I'm in complete control of everything, and therefore I can handle anything, including heroin. For whatever reason and for however long it builds up in my head, I've gone and used. It was especially true when our offices were at Kings Cross and the scene was right outside the window, on the streets. There were occasions when I felt lonely, as if it was give, give, give, and where was the littlest bit of pleasure for me? I would sit at home every night after work and, particularly when I was finding it impossible to sleep, I'd think about getting a bit of gear, because it helped me through the night. I used through a particular bad time when every day for a week I went bang out, bang out. But it cost me £500 and when you're not earning illegally, you can't do it on your salary. That time it was clear-cut depression, a case of thinking as long as I was dying anyway, I might as well die happily.

I won't pretend heroin wasn't an integral part of my life for a long time. It was my life for over ten years. To be honest, I enjoyed it. There is no other drug, including alcohol, that can ever give me the same satisfaction as heroin. I've been scripted for methadone for five years. People can be on methadone scripts and live a life as normally as the next person. No one would look at me and think she's on methadone, not anybody who's looking at me as the director of Positively Women. The amount of methadone you take makes a difference - I'm on only ten milligrams. My script is not just about my drug addiction, it's also about pain control. If I'm having a lot of pain in my joints I have an extra tablet. Why suffer when there's something there to help?

During the last five years I've become so much more accepting about who I am, what I am, and towards my attitudes and feelings. I have the confidence to believe that no one else is necessarily right or has the answers I need. I believe I was meant to be doing this work. I believe I was meant to have Laura. I believe the hard years of my relationship with my parents, had a purpose, because recently it's become so good and close. Life is about getting the right balance; from the amount of coffee you drink, to the amount of support you need, to what you can offer and expect from friends. I believe that my power is within myself and that it's something that everyone has inside them. My spirituality is very much for me and is about keeping my sanity in this absolutely crazy world. It's not a side of me people expect. The strong political woman fighting for women's rights and standing up for what she believes in is a true part of me, but it hurts me when people have an image of me as a hard woman, because I'm also a sensitive, perceptive person.

I have only ever had three serious relationships with men. There was my first boyfriend, Gary, and then Mario for ten years, and finally Laura's father, Robert, who I was with for two years. Although he wasn't physically violent he had the same traits as Mario. I kidded myself about what I was looking for in a man. I always went for tall, big men; I was definitely looking for a protector, somebody who could put his big strong arms around me and say, 'There, there, Sheila, it's all right. I'll look after you, I'll take the responsibility. You just stay safe in my arms.' That's always been my romantic fantasy of a relationship, but do I even need to say what a load of crap that is? Because basically it was my little arms holding the man!

With Robert, I was the decision-maker, I was the personality. I was attracted to him because I thought this man is so quiet and deep, there must be a lot more in there and I was going to find it. But when I got there, there was nothing. I should be angry about Robert because he's been irresponsible about Laura, never giving me any money, turning up when he feels like it. But I can't even feel anger towards him. I just think he's pathetic and I even feel sorry for him.

I've been celibate for over three years. I've had no wish at all to go into a relationship. I never even feel any sexual stirring. I used to enjoy masturbation, but I don't even do that now. It could be virus connected, but I also think it's a hell of a lot more. My fear isn't about being with a man and telling him he's got to wear a condom. I have no problem around that. The man I sleep with would know about me and would hopefully be right-on enough to wear one. I'm so much my own person now, and I've got such a nice set up with my daughter and my work, that for a start to contemplate sharing her and the rest of my life as it now is with anyone else would take a lot.

My needs are filled by close friends now. I'm not hetero-sexual and I'm not lesbian. I'm celibate and that's my sexual-ity. If I clicked with someone of either sex it would be fine with me, but I would tread very carefully. I like what lots of lesbi-ans have: I envy the closeness, the bond, the night-out for lesbians. Heterosexual women don't have all that. I also feel a wee bit left out because I'm not included in the lesbian scene. But I also understand the specialness of people identifying to-gether, supporting each other - if I walk into a room full of positive women there's a bonding, a spark.

Of course there are times when I go to bed and think it would be nice to have someone to cuddle up to. But it would have to be on my terms. I put my daughter to bed in her little room and she's sweet and warm and secure. Then I go up to my own bed and I lay there in my room and snuggle up and think, there's Laura and me and it's fine.

There are quite a few lesbians working in the AIDS field, doing good work. From what I see within the lesbian scene no one admits they're sleeping with men or using drugs, because they're such taboo subjects. It's very difficult to weigh up how many lesbians use drugs because your sexuality becomes rela-tively unimportant when you're using heroin. When I was in the drug scene I might have known a woman for years and not been aware of whether she was a lesbian or not. I wasn't in-terested in their sexuality, I was interested in either selling or buying heroin off them. The reality is that I've shared with lesbian heroin users in the past. All the taboos mean there are some lesbians around who are not being very honest about things they do which might relate to HIV transmission.

It's as important for heterosexual women to have discussions and information about HIV. Straight women are not all the same - they differ from each other and have different identities. At Positively Women we try to speak about all these issues be-cause in sexual matters, it's about coming to terms with feel-ings around a variety of sexual practices. Personally I'm not interested in anybody's intimate goings on in bed but we have to open up discussions so that safer sex practices make sense to everyone. It's no good making assumptions about what women do or don't do sexually.

I know condoms are not widely used. I get feedback from friends and read the literature. A friend of mine lives with a guy and they go to a pub which is very heterosexual. AIDS is not being taken on by the people in that pub; it's hardly talked about. If it does come up, it's in a gossipy, negative way - it's always someone else's problem. These men have the 'All right Tracy, you've got a pack of condoms! You must be looking for someone tonight' attitude. Sometimes I'm tempted to give up trying to educate people on safer sex because so many won't take it on. They don't realize the pain and only see it as others' problem or possibility.

Having said all that I admit that Robert and I didn't have safe sex. Life, and often sexuality in particular, is not always straightforward. We have certainties, but we have ambivalences, and confusions too. Robert knew about me - I told him about my status and asked him to use a condom I had with me the first time we had sex. But he didn't want to use one. I could have refused to have sex with him, but I could only take so much responsibility. I think there were two reasons why he refused and why I let him. One was to do with a lack of realization on his part of the reality of HIV, even though he knew the facts and was aware of the risks. I think he did it as a token of his love for me - he loved me so much that he didn't mind getting the virus. He wanted to be with me and was willing to share everything with me, HIV included. Secondly, I think he believed it might seem like a rejection of me. If I'm honest (and I think all of us who are HIV positive have to honest about these things because they are so complex) I might have felt a tiny bit of rejection from him if he wouldn't touch me without a condom on. That ambivalence allowed me to push common sense aside. None of it is an excuse for not practising safer sex, only an attempt to understand why I (and others) don't always do what we believe in.

Thankfully, Robert wasn't positive after all that time. Statistics indicate that the virus may be transmitted during a first exposure, but on the other hand, you could sleep with someone positive for five years with a 25 to 35 per cent chance of transmission. You can never predict. You don't know if it's going to be you, or your neighbour, or your sister or brother. It also appears that a positive man can more easily transmit the virus to a woman through vaginal penetration, rather than the other way round. Magic Johnson's HIV status has focused much needed attention on heterosexual HIV, but it's a shame that the danger to women from unsafe sex with HIV positive men is being overlooked. Women are being put in the role of dangerous people men have to watch out for.

There are different strains of HIV virus and you can be positive already and then be reinfected with a different sort of HIV. Two viruses getting together may form something else, something stronger perhaps. Also, if your immune system is suppressed, you have to be careful about any sort of infection, including other STDs (Sexually Transmitted Diseases). When two positive people live together they may think it's great, no more necessity for safer sex. But that's not true. I've got my own virus, I certainly wouldn't want anyone else's.

I've gone through a time where I felt I'd got it together about my status and around dying. But just lately because I've had PCP (pneumocystis carinii pneumonia) again, it's all brought it flooding back. When you're well, especially for someone like me who works in the AIDS field, you're there for other people and on some levels you tend to forget about being positive yourself. So when I got ill with PCP recently, I thought this is what AIDS is about. You hear such terrible stories about everyone else, but if you're not going through it yourself, even if you're positive, it's hard to relate to.

I got depressed when I was ill this time. My first thought was for my daughter Laura and what would happen to her if I wasn't here. I always thought she would go to my sister and family in Scotland as there was something about going to my family that felt warm and secure. I thought a lot about work too. I'm sure everyone goes through this who has serious ill-health. Should I be working full-time? Should I be cutting down? Can I afford it financially? If I only have a couple of years to live should I be spending more time with Laura?

Then I thought about my death. I've always thought I was a special person and that somehow death wasn't going to happen to me in the near future, but the reality is that it may. Having PCP the second time slotted things into place a bit: I wasn't so special and such a crusader for women and AIDS that death could be warded off indefinitely. When illness hit home I re-alized that my body's been through so much that in reality I could be dead in six months, two years, or whenever.

Even in illness there are light moments. I was in the hospi-tal waiting in the clinic a while ago - I usually don't chat with anyone else about symptoms but I met this woman, she called herself a transvestite, and we got talking about AIDS in gen-eral, about how long we'd have to wait, and finally we got onto the subject of T-cells (a low count indicates a decline in im-munity) and what our counts were. I told her mine was quite low at sixteen, and she replied that hers was much lower at only four. Then she told me how she wakes up in the morning and gives her T-cells names and mentally encourages them to mate and have lots and lots of babies. I responded by telling her that because I've got sixteen, when I get a pain in my back I know they're holding a support group. We laughed. It was so nice that we could sit and talk in this way, making light of it all.

When I think about death, it's not about fear - because al-though I've not actually lived with death (and I know that sounds really gory), I have a lot to do with it. I have no fear of dying. (Well not too much anyway!?!) It's more to do with the people you leave behind, and about leaving Laura in particular. I try to avoid thinking about it because I get such a knotted pain inside. As much as I know she's going to be loved and cared for, it's not the same as having a mum there. Oh god, what would she do?

I never regret having her. I'd still go through with it. I've never ever experienced giving somebody love like you do to your child. It's an absolute joy, the best thing I've ever bloody done in my life. After all the shit I've gone through, all the shit I've created for myself and others, I feel I've done something really positive and worthwhile. I'm crying even now writing this, I love her so much. It would be better if I were around for more of her life but she's lovely, she's a beautiful wee girl, she's happy, content, very secure. I had my daughter Laura after believing it wasn't possible because I was positive. At the time all the doctors and all the odds they quoted said that the two of us would be dead in three months. But we went through the pregnancy successfully and she is now three, HIV negative, and a great thriving little girl.

Laura's nursery doesn't know about my personal situation. I told the woman who runs it what I do and where I work, and I even gave her one of our cards - the reality is that she may come across a child who is positive and she should have information if that situation arises. She was quite open about it. Laura is negative; if she were positive it would be an issue for Laura herself. For instance, if she was getting extra tired compared to other children it might be related to her positive status. No one would think twice about informing a school that their child was diabetic or asthmatic, or had sickle cell because these are accepted, if difficult, conditions, but because of the stigma which exists around AIDS, it's much more difficult to consider divulging information.

I'm careful not to advise women to tell social services or schools about their status. I try to educate around possibilities and support women in whatever choices they make, rather than telling them what they should do. That could be dangerous. If they told a school, for instance, and it didn't work out, there might be a lot of anger and blame which could be directed at Positively Women. I could handle it if the woman came back and spoke to me about how she felt, but the odds are that she wouldn't get in touch again. After the pros and cons have been fully explained, the choice must come from the woman herself and be related to her experience.

Since having Laura, I've had quite a few illnesses. There is no hard evidence about the effect of pregnancy on HIV positive women. The current thinking on the risk of a woman passing on HIV to her unborn baby is anything from 15 to 30 per cent. But because I wasn't in great health anyway, the pregnancy did have a negative effect on my body, although I've never had a moment's regret about that.

Positively Women is worthwhile but it's a different kind of achievement. I'm too tired to live up to the superwoman/heroine role. I put a lot of energy into the challenge of building up the organization. It started from nothing and now Princess Di has launched our new headquarters. It's running and will run with or without me. Yes, I'd be sorely missed and I know that I'm strongly identified with Positively Women. Lately, though, I think my job is done. This may sound a bit dramatic but really, I can't work full-time any more; I'm just not healthy enough. Also it isn't the same, the challenge is gone. Basically now it's about going in and doing a day's work. I was happier when I was getting no salary, and it was running from my house. Now I've got the director's label, a big office, and a salary, it's just not the same. If I had my health I might leave and work around something else I feel strongly about.

I get through the bad times by talking to friends and doing a lot of crying and thinking of Laura. I try to apply my knowledge of what others in crisis need to myself, but sometimes I'm not altogether successful. I may not have a group to go to but I have got good supportive friends and they mean the world to me.

There are many observations I could make about HIV and AIDS - things which go beyond Positively Women. At times I think, yes, Positively Women is important by anybody's standards, but at other times I get cynical and think people accept us because HIV and AIDS is just another issue banging on the door. I feel patronized by the government and social services who play such a big part in people's lives when they're in crisis. They're so powerful and closed. If you don't have a social work degree behind you, you're not accepted, yet traditional social work attitudes are being questioned more and more these days.

Sometimes I try to stop myself thinking about AIDS on a world basis, because it gets beyond my comprehension - what's happening in Africa, in the Hispanic and black communities in America, in the Philippines, which countries are recognizing it, which ones are denying it. If the British government accepts that HIV is an condition you cannot catch through hugging and kissing, how come another government in another part of the world is putting HIV positive people in prison until a cure is found? It confuses me. What communication is going on with between the world's governments?

In every social issue you have to have militants, the dedicated politicos who will lead the way for others. But I don't like it if militants take up an issue simply for the sake of it, whether they're affected by it or not, or if something is made political for someone else's ends. I've always believed in making a stand and I believe it's important that people affected by AIDS are not seen as passive. I would rather see people with AIDS and HIV leading the way. The government cannot be allowed to make decisions which may be against our interests. I'm getting involved now in the United Kingdom Declaration of Human Rights for People with HIV and AIDS. That's the sort of politics I believe will be effective. The gay community has received recognition and reclaimed a lot of power through their reaction to the AIDS crisis. But I'm coming from being a woman, a single parent, and an ex-drug user. I'm involved in trying to run a women's organization with services, where previously there were very few. We have had to take on board the relative invisibility of women who are HIV positive or have AIDS and to recognize their different needs. I work towards achieving physical and mental balance in my life and that's connected to the sort of political involvement I chose to make.

In my opinion Positively Women has got through to more people about women's issues than any other AIDS organization. Quietly, we have changed a lot and women with HIV and AIDS are finally being recognized.

SHEILA'S DIARY

Written just after being back in hospital
with PCP in early 1991.

Where do I begin tonight? I went off to bed early because Laura was being a pain and when I eventually got her to bed she managed to climb out and come in to me feeling very pleased with herself and with an air that it was natural for her to do an assault course over her cot. So we snuggled up for another hour, I took a couple of sleeping tablets and she fell asleep, I didn't! I got up feeling as if I wanted to do something creative, so I put a few photos in the Liberty photo holder I'd been given as a gift, filled up my folder with blank paper so I could write down feelings and ideas as they came up. It's going to be a help in sorting my life out and, oh god, does it need sorting out.

I've been down just lately. I suppose my illness has something to do with it, but there are so many other things that I don't feel strong enough to cope with. I found out a long time ago that people will feel sympathetic for so long - when they see you on your feet even though inside your body may be feeling as weak as shit, they begin to feel resentful that you're not in there doing your bit. I am thoroughly down at the moment - anything I have I give to Laura and I feel I do a pretty good job at that although I never have any one to compare to so I never quite know.

My two big problems are, am I going to be healthy enough to go back and do a good job at Positively Women or will I make myself even iller by going back? Also I am in about eight to ten thousand pounds debt which is just about doing me in because I'm not managing as it is on what I'm earning.

It breaks my heart that I haven't the energy to do everything with Laura all the time. She's a big girl and even to swing her round just about does me in. I don't feel sorry for myself or at least I hope I don't come over like that, I just want strength and energy and from that I could get a bit of positive thinking back. There are so many things I want to write about. I hope anyone reading this isn't too confused and can make connections. The sleeping tablets are working now, so soon it's off to sleep.

You know I went to the hospital today and got my usual check over, blood taken, went on the nebulizer for the pentamidine which helps keep PCP away! I've been off AZT for one month and was meant to start DDi today but it hadn't arrived, so I'll start Monday. I'm pretty scared about it - okay it may be great but it may give me horrific side-effects and then how will I look after Laura? All I want is to get myself organized and be a good mum, a fun mum, not one she's always seeing lying in a hospital bed. I know now after another heavy talk with my parents that Laura will be brought up beautifully and even if they are a little naughty with their politics. They were with me too and I sorted mine out - she's had a good start. I'm sleepy now - hope I will keep jotting down everything so it comes out as natural and honest as possible.

Later... I'm back again and feeling a little more organized tonight. I've been cleaning, tidying, washing, ironing and getting the house shipshape. I'm one of those people who finds it hard to have a tidy mind if my house isn't tidy. So tonight it's getting there and I now need to sort out my paper work and lots of other bits and pieces. I promised myself that I would dedicate a little time every now and then for writing.

The phone just rang and it was my friend Allison - she is a good friend and yet when she rang to see how I was, all I felt was anger towards her, as if how dare she be away for two weeks enjoying herself and not be here with me. I even lowered my voice a little and talked slower just so she got the message I was depressed. Why do I do that, how dare I, what do I expect from friends? If it wasn't for them I would really be in the shit, looking after Laura all the time. God, I don't want to be like that; it seems to be going into months that I have felt either ill, weak, tired, depressed, oh, and everything else. People must be well fed up with me. I know it's not all my fault but I sometimes feel I could at least speak more cheerfully and then it may help change things.

Still later... It's now 17 February and no, I didn't get any Valentines from anyone - either sex - but I can live with that. My life has taken another turn and I don't know if it's the passing of time, or the DDi (Did you know there are only me and another 219 people on this in the whole of Britain!), but I'm feeling better. I just read over what I had written before and thought, what crap - a bit of Temazepan Twaddle! Life is okay but it always is when I have my health back. I'm working full-time and getting lots done, I'm having fun with Laura and our relationship goes from strength to strength - unlike my spelling. My home is clean and tidy and cosy which is important to me. Mind you, my mother was over the top about cleanliness in the house. We used to call her Howard (as in Hughes) and I think I have picked up a bit of her fanatical behaviour. I don't mind Laura drawing on the walls as long as she does it neatly! Friends have been dropping by and really I've been having quite an all right time.

I did go through a couple of days when I couldn't keep my eyes open. I call it my virus tiredness because it doesn't matter if I've done a lot or not, I still have no control over keeping my eyes open. This frightens me a little but also pisses me off. I had a bit of a blow out with a friend who is used to this sort of thing with me, and I just started crying and telling her how I was fed up having AIDS, pissed off with hospitals, pissed off with having to take pills at certain times every day of my fucking life, pissed off with having to hide the truth to half the people I meet, fucked off with fighting for the rights

of women with AIDS when I know half the world have the attitude that we're no better than a piece of shit. Phew! But I
also know that I've got a lot of respect in the AIDS field, a lot
of people really care about me.

But Jesus, people in the Gulf are getting their brains blown
out, children are dying in their hundreds every day of starva-
tion, sexual abuse, rape, I could go on and on, and what I'm
doing feels so bloody pointless, life seems so stupid, the world
seems absolutely fucking crazy - not seems - IS. But after all
that I know I have to make the best of my own life and I love
Laura so much that I do a lot of it for her. I know I need to
feel these things and get them out of my system but sometimes....
Anyway if I just get on living my life with Laura and helping
women live theirs a little better sometimes, it works out all right
and it makes me happy.

Religion has always fascinated me and I've had some different experiences around it, but my favourite words for years,
which I love and try to live by are: Grant me the serenity to
accept the things I cannot change, the courage to change the
things I can, and the wisdom to know the difference.

I'm closing now to watch French and Saunders on the telly.

DECEMBER 1991
I want to leave you with something really positive. It's 10
December, my daughter has just turned three. Tonight we're
putting up the Christmas tree (one that can be replanted for next
year of course - rain forest and all that).

Anyway, I'm not finished yet.... God, that sounds like a threat!

SUSAN

Susan is a thirty-two year old black
African, who was diagnosed HIV positive
in July 1987 and as having AIDS in
August 1990.
Her daughter is nearly two years old
and is HIV negative.

1989

IT ALL STARTEDlike this: I was a bit disappointed about
the way my boyfriend was behaving and I thought it was best
to make a clean break. I decided to have an AIDS test; I wasn't
sure about whether I had it or not, but I had my suspicions. I
knew it would mean a lot of things, like not having kids, so I
thought the best thing was to find out. I went to the hospital
and talked to a doctor who asked me why I wanted the test.
He asked if I'd ever had a bisexual boyfriend or taken drugs -
and I answered no. He asked if I'd ever been a prostitute and
again I answered no. Then he went on to say I looked fine and
that he didn't think I needed to take the test. I explained that I
came from Central Africa and that I might have it, who knows?
So I took the test and was told to come back in two week's
time. Even though I was worried, after the way he talked to
me I didn't believe I had it.

When I returned to the hospital they kept me waiting for so
long - was my file lost? I started worrying. I can still feel the
feeling now, stomach churning. I said, 'What's wrong, why
are these people not showing me the results?' Eventually they
called me in and the doctor said it was bad, bad news. From
that time onwards I felt like I was in a dream; as if somebody
was talking to me from a long way away. I don't remember a

37

word he said. I do remember that he finally took me to the health adviser and she told me more about it. That's when I really started realizing all the things it meant.

I always wanted to have kids, so that was the first thing to strike me. I'd never really had a family; my mother was okay, but when my stepfather arrived I had problems and never again felt it was my family. I thought that if I had my own kids it would make a difference. I felt so bad that day in the hospital; I cried out, 'I'll never have a family? Never get married? Never have kids?' I broke down and cried and cried and cried. I was repeating the same words '...very sad ...very sad ...very sad'. The woman who talked to me was supportive and even now she's my friend. We've even gone out a couple of times for a drink.

I don't know how I got it. I don't even know how long I've had it. Once when I was travelling in my country I had a high fever and had to have an injection; at that time I didn't have a partner. I don't know - maybe I had it from before that from a partner. I don't really know. So perhaps I got it sexually, but I can't be sure. In a way there's no point in trying to find out and anyway it would be very difficult because I can't go with my little list asking people to go have and test and see whether they have AIDS or not. Socially that would mean my life would be finished.

I've never told anybody. Sometimes I get depressed, but still I've never talked to anyone from my country about it, not even my parents. I know if I did, too many other people would get to know about it. Unlike other conditions, you can't tell about HIV, so it can stay a secret. People here are prejudiced about AIDS; they think you are promiscuous and that's why you got it in the first place. It's the same in my country, even worse, because people are ignorant about the whole subject. They think you are a leper or something; they wouldn't come near you, wouldn't drink a cup of tea in your place because they believe they could get the virus that way. I would be very, very miserable. That's why I haven't even told my previous partner.

What I've found out is that most women I know who have the virus have slept with a man; it seems it's more difficult for a woman to give it to a man than the other way round. But men will start talking about you and say, 'That girl has got AIDS'. They don't say you have HIV, because to them there is no difference between it and AIDS. Then you find you are an outcast. I get so angry I can't talk about it - sometimes when I'm sitting on a train or in a bus I feel like shouting aloud because I'm so frustrated. Even when I'm with my friends at a party, I break down and cry. I look at all the people and think how they don't know I have the virus and how miserable it makes me that I can't tell them. Maybe they would understand, I don't know for sure, but I can't risk it, you see. It's better not to because rejection is the worst thing that could ever happen to anyone in this situation, it can destroy you completely. But it means your friends don't understand a lot of your life.

When I'm with people who have the virus they don't feel sorry for me and I don't feel sorry for them. Although we give each other support, that's all, because we're in the same boat, aren't we? The last thing I want is sympathy - all I need is understanding. Being able to go along to Positively Women has been very helpful because I can relate to the women there and they can understand how I feel even if I don't say much.

Only a person who knows people who have the virus, and has intimately discussed things with them, can really understand. There are times when you just feel so sad and miserable, so angry with yourself and with the whole world, times when you start thinking of everything you've done in your life. You don't regret your life, but you wonder if you hadn't done a particular thing, like been in a certain place, this wouldn't have happened. It's like death, when somebody dies, and you start regretting when nothing can be changed. Whereas really, you'd probably have done the same things even if you knew what you now know.

Being HIV positive has changed me a lot. I'm a much nicer person than I used to be. Although I know that we are all going to die one day, the fact that you have the virus means there is a bigger threat of death being nearer than you expected. When you don't have any problems you just feel well, you don't think that it might end tomorrow. Now I think in terms of years; sometimes I give myself three years, five years, who knows?

It also makes relationships with men difficult. To tell the truth I don't think it would be easy for me unless I got a boy-friend who was also positive. Even if a man loved you that much, which I doubt, most men, in my country anyway, wouldn't really understand and sacrifice their fear of being infected. It's a pipe-dream. I have a friend who says that she doesn't want to have friends who are HIV positive, she wants someone who is healthy. But that's not the way I see it. I know if you're in a relationship with someone who is also positive, you have a fear that one of you is going to leave, but at the same time you give each other confidence and strength. I don't see how a person who isn't positive can really give you strength or support.

I haven't had sex for a very long time, since I split up with my previous boyfriend because... I can't... I can't. First of all I wouldn't have sex with someone I didn't love; even if I had it for physical needs, I think I would feel guilty and uptight after. It's the fear of giving somebody the virus. With love-making you have to kiss and cuddle, you do all those things, and then there is penetration. If you practise safer sex you can protect by using a condom, but what about kissing? I know there's no reason why you should be able to catch the virus from kissing - I've heard that to pass it by kissing you would have to drink two pints of someone's saliva, but there's still the fear, the worry, which makes you lose confidence. And also I would have a big dark secret.

Recently I met someone who is very interested in me and who seems very understanding. I'm attracted to him but I feel I have a responsibility to tell him. If I don't want to tell him, it means I can't have an affair with him. If I do tell him maybe I'll be rejected which would hurt me more than anything else. I want to go on living and enjoying myself but I'm not sure how.

My attitude towards everything in life has changed. I understand people better now; I don't judge them as I used to do. When people judge me I feel very angry; usually I'm stubborn and I show it. I believe we should all learn from and understand other people. I'll give you an example: by my own moral standards, I wouldn't really approve of gay men or lesbians, but that is my own opinion, it doesn't go further than that. I am not them, so I don't even know how they feel. I don't know how they started or all their life history. How can I say it's bad? I can't. You look at the rest of the world and you read in the paper that gay people asked for AIDS. They didn't! When they do penetrative sex they can get bruised, whereas for a woman it's not that easy. I've heard that gay men used to have a lot of communal sex but then you can't blame them. I think the reason they had that kind of sex is because they were rejected by society. I'd like to know more gay people who are HIV positive or have AIDS. I'd like to understand how they feel and cope. Maybe there are gay men and lesbians in my country but I never came in contact with them, so I still wonder what goes on, what happens between them?

I don't dread going to the hospital; I like going, even for a chat. They really care about you and sometimes I think people with the virus get more attention than any other patients. Recently I had a smear test and they found abnormal cells. I only had to wait one month for an appointment for laser treatment, whereas for anyone else it would have been six. But sometimes they don't have the answers for every one of your questions. Most of all, you don't have to lie about AIDS, which is a relief.

Most of my friends are very broad-minded and I think they probably see AIDS as I do. My friends don't laugh about it, they say it's a serious thing. One of them told me recently, 'Who knows, I may have AIDS, but I wont go for a test because I don't want to know.' At the same time, I know if I told a friend, eventually everyone would know and the information could easily fall on the wrong ears.

The most important thing to understand is that when you are part of a community, and most of my friends are from the same community, your life is different from most people's in this country. We in Africa are not like people are here where individualism is very important and if you have a problem, it's yours and you don't share it with anyone. The attitude is different in our community. We share a lot and sometimes it's good to do that. But also our worst fear is being rejected by our community. It's hard to explain, but because the community is so important to me, my fear of rejection is probably greater than an English person's would be.

In Africa people are so frightened of AIDS. Most people must have got it sexually or though medical injections, but people don't know this. We had a Minister who said, 'Love carefully', which meant that AIDS was only a sexual problem, nothing else. Of course he was referring to heterosexual sex because in Africa AIDS is not associated with a gay community. Not many people take drugs in my country either - heroin and things like that. Although they say sex is the main problem, I think it's more to do with injections with unsterilized needles. We don't have enough needles so they are often re-used. In this country AIDS has been more common for gay men, but that doesn't mean heterosexual men don't have it. In my clinic I'm surprised by how many heterosexual men, even married ones, have it. I wonder how they got it?

The virus has set me free in a way: I am now more important to myself than before. If I want to do something, I do it. If I don't want to, nobody's going to force me to. And if somebody feels that I should have done something, too bad, I get angry and I show it; it's my own way of coping.

I think women have different experiences of having the virus than men. For example, most gay men wouldn't dream of having children, whereas most woman want to be married and have kids. You might get married if you are HIV positive, but you know you'll never have kids. If you're a positive and get pregnant, there's a risk to your health as well as the baby's. If the baby was born ill and died it would be much sadder than not having one at all. It's so painful to think about. You have to be realistic but it doesn't stop you wanting a child.

There's a common attitude that if you're an HIV positive woman it's because you've been promiscuous. This bothers me a lot. People think men can be promiscuous and women can't, but to me it's all the same. Why is it wrong for a woman to have strong sexual desires and not for a man? I wouldn't tolerate a promiscuous man; I would expect the same of a man as I would of a woman. Most heterosexuals, men and women, think they are safe from HIV but I know they aren't. It's been proved that there are many who are positive - and there may be others who have the virus and don't know it. A woman has a boyfriend - neither of them is what you would call promiscuous but perhaps he has sex with another woman one day, comes down with an STD, and infects the first woman. It doesn't mean he's guilty of anything. The only people I can say are guilty are the ones who set about to do it intentionally. Even those people I'm not sure about because sometimes people get angry... at society for instance. For others it may be their only way of coping and they may be denying to themselves that they are doing anything dangerous.

The future only scares me when I get an illness or infection, no matter how small. That's when I get paranoid and fear I'm going to die. But when I'm all right I don't waste my time thinking about it. A work colleague of mine and I were discussing AIDS and she told me she was scared. She said, 'You know, this virus is so scary and even now I don't know whether I have it or not.' It was all imagined, she didn't have it. But she woke up one morning, took her kids to school and had a car accident in which she died instantly. When I think about her, I say to myself, who am I to start worrying about dying?

What worries me most is being ill or helpless. You start looking at people, wondering what they would think if you died, what they would say? I have a feeling that if I get AIDS and see that it's getting out of control or that I'm not going to survive, I'll have to do something about it.

I have hopes that they may find a drug to contain AIDS. Not to cure, because I think viruses are not curable. All I can say to myself is look after yourself. I used to enjoy eating and never worried about what I ate, but these days I have to. Now I have to count every gram of fibre and it takes away the pleasure of food. For instance, every morning I eat Weetabix which I never used to like, but because I know it's high in fibre I eat it.

1991

Sarah, my daughter, is now over a year old. Two years ago I didn't believe I would ever have a child, but then there was very little information about HIV positive women having children and most of it was negative. I was told it was a risk to my life and that the child might also be positive and I didn't want to risk losing a child or my health. Two years ago I didn't have a boyfriend which made the possibility of having a child even more remote.

Since then I read as much information as I could about positive women who had children; I also met a few positive women who had chosen to have children. I was especially moved by one woman I was close to who went ahead and had a child who is now over two years old and perfectly healthy. That woman was not in very good health at the time and I feared she wouldn't survive the pregnancy, but she did and it was like a miracle. At the time I had a boyfriend and health-wise I was in good condition, so it felt like my only chance. Who knows, my health might deteriorate at some future stage and then it would be more difficult to make a decision. As my partner wanted a child as well, I felt it was the right time.

My partner, who I have now split with, is not positive. We were sleeping together, generally using safe sex, but not always. That's how I got pregnant. After that we never had unsafe sex and when I was seven months pregnant he had a test which was negative. After that, he tested again and was still negative. Our relationship was good in many ways. To tell the truth, I didn't tell him I was positive at first, but eventually when I did, at first he was supportive, although some bitterness came later. In the beginning he was in some kind of shock which kept him from reacting. I tried to talk to him about it and I also asked him to have a test which he refused to do, probably because he was scared. Even when he had the test things didn't get better between us because he couldn't cope with the fact that I was positive. Our life was in shambles for a while although we stayed together for a certain time. I wanted him to go for help, to talk to other people and try to come to terms with my status but he couldn't bring himself to do it.

We're not from the same tribe, or the same background, which created a problem for my family. At the end of the day I told my parents it was my life, if I lived with him it was what I wanted to do and they couldn't stop me. But their hostility sometimes made me feel frantic and sad - I could always sense it and it created tension. However, it never bothered either of us as much as the fact that I was positive. He failed to come to terms with that. I realize now that we never talked as much as we should have. I used to try to ask him how he felt and get him to talk to me. I wouldn't have minded if he told me he was scared or even that he hated me, but he never did. Ultimately I said that if we never went through that process at home, we could never really get on. It's a shame because he was good for me and we were good friends, but we never talked about the most important thing affecting our lives and that ended the relationship.

What made it so difficult for him was probably the thought that at some stage I would get ill and die; he couldn't cope with those thoughts. He felt I wouldn't be able to give him all the things he wanted in life, like a lifelong partnership, companionship, making future plans. Also he wanted more children and perhaps he thought he would be better off with another woman. At least we talked about not having any more children and at one stage we agreed we should stop our relationship so he could try to live with somebody else he would be able to have more children with, as well as a more certain future. He couldn't decide about it - some times he couldn't live without me for a minute and then he'd wonder. He was angry about the whole situation. Eventually, when we decided to split up, it was more like an excuse and I finally decided I couldn't cope with the continuous uncertainty in our relationship. It brought up too much stress. Since we finished completely, I haven't looked back. Unless he comes to terms with my illness and says that whatever my life is, short or long, it's enough for him, we will never get back together. Anyway, I don't think that's possible now because I feel more comfortable without him. I have met new friends who are positive; I've found out that at times I need to be with them and to talk with them about my feelings. They have helped me come to terms with my life.

When I was pregnant I had no problems until I gave birth. I believe the reason my health deteriorated then is because of the emotional stress I was going through, plus the work of coping with a baby. When I first had the baby, my partner and I were not on good terms. We'd had a row and for three months he didn't see me or help so I ended up coping on my own which was traumatic. My health suffered but I still don't think it was caused by the pregnancy or birth. I had to do all the physical things virtually by myself - the washing, looking after her, all the cooking. At home, usually when you have given birth you don't have to do anything except feed the baby. Here, sometimes I'm too tired to eat, too tired to do anything and I'm with the baby twenty-four hours a day. The only time I have been away from her was when she was six months old, but before that it was never for even an hour.

At home everything is done for you by your family. You wake up in the morning and they help you with the washing up and look after you and the baby. This goes on for anything from three months to six months - it's that long before you start doing any physical work. It made me miss my family a lot because I think of all the things my relatives would have done for me which nobody else can do. People here are busy most of the time. As much as they'd like to help, or do, it's not enough

- you always need more than they can give you. At home there are so many people who have the time. Consequently you recover very quickly. I had chronic back pain when Sarah was five months old and even now I have it because of the physical work I do.

For most of the time I've known I was positive, I never told anyone - my family, or my community. It created great stress not to tell and sometimes I wanted to so badly. But then I got PCP and was in hospital for two weeks; while I was there I thought about it a lot. That was when the doctors told me I had AIDS and I decided it was time to tell a few people I was positive. So I told two of my best friends in London and then I wrote to my mother. Her reaction was as I expected and was why I didn't want to tell her in the first place - she was very worried I was going to die. Although she wanted to come and see me, I began to think of going there instead, in order to see the rest of my family. I'm close to my sisters and brother; I haven't told them yet but I might. After that I didn't really mind other people knowing I was positive so much. I won't ever go out and announce it, but if they find out about it, it no longer bothers me. Once, after I'd been in the hospital, I was asked to talk to someone else who was positive and I refused. I was scared they might tell someone else about me. But now, after having Sarah, and having received some support from my ex-partner, as well as knowing other people who accept me, I have more confidence. Those changes in my life have given me the faith and courage to face difficult things and I have discovered that once you start talking to other people from your own nationality, you sometimes find they have the same fears about the community that you have. It makes you stronger to realize your common bond. In the past I had positive friends but they came from other communities. Now I find if I give something of myself to people who are as scared as I was before, it helps them feel more relaxed and relieves some of their worries. It makes me feel good to think I've helped someone sort themselves out.

The whole idea of community is complicated by the fact that we may be from different nationalities and be divided among ourselves. However, I find that in general, women who are positive seem to get along well, no matter what their nationality is. In my experience, we have always come out with a positive attitude towards each other - they are convinced I care about them, and I believe they care about me. Contrary to all my fears, I have never experienced rejection. Maybe they talk about me behind my back, who knows? But so many people are dying within my community that everyone is scared and people are much more understanding. The way they talk about people with AIDS has changed. Before there was a lot of hostility and they wouldn't go near a person who had AIDS, or they would say things like, 'Can you imagine, I drank from her cup.' Now they tend to be more knowledgeable and you never hear such things - you can get into a heated argument about it, you can score points and end up making the person think it's not as bad as they thought it was.

I think safer sex information for different cultures is important because it's necessary to understand that different nationalities have different sexual practices. For example, in my own culture you wouldn't talk about masturbation but in another culture both women and men masturbate. Many people from my country would find it strange that a man or a woman could masturbate in bed together. However, it's difficult to imagine separate pamphlets for every single different group. As I said, even in my country there are different nationalities, different languages, different sexual practice, different cultures altogether. How can you really satisfy the needs of everyone?

But people are becoming more aware. You will find that some of the so-called sexual taboos are breaking down. For instance, people from my nationality are not supposed to practise oral sex. But people do it. I talk to many of them who tell me they have oral sex, so things are changing and there's no point in being dogmatic about sexual practices. For some people homosexuality was a taboo, and still is, but I know now that there are homosexuals in my country. Many people still find it difficult to come to terms with the fact that it exists but now it is not so surprising if somebody is a homosexual. People might not like it but they wouldn't simply hurl abuse as they used to; attitudes are changing.

In my country sometimes people who come from a certain area are blamed for causing AIDS. But people have had to realize it isn't only coming from one area. The people from the north used to say that AIDS was especially prevalent in the south; others used to say it was caused by witchcraft. However, now almost all families have been affected by AIDS. It used to be something distant, something that would never reach you, but in the last two or three years so many people have died of AIDS - including stars and top people - that everyone from the poorest to the richest has been touched. That reality, more than anything else, has changed attitudes towards people with AIDS.

I wonder what will happen in this country? People are not as in touch with each other as we are in many African countries. I may live here and have neighbours, but I never really know the people who live around me; I can spend months without seeing my next door neighbour. Unless you move within a community it is difficult to talk about the virus. Ex-drug users, gay people, I think they can find people to talk to more easily; they tend to communicate through common interests. For heterosexuals there is a lot of hypocrisy and difficulty. I've met women who tell me that their husband doesn't want anyone to know or that he doesn't want her to talk to anybody about it. I can't imagine many heterosexuals talking openly about their son who was positive. Positive people get together in groups because they're positive; they tend not to talk to other people about living with HIV, usually because they're frightened to. But if those people who aren't positive knew there were large numbers of positive people it might get them thinking. If we didn't have to hide, we wouldn't remain faceless. No one could continue to think it's a gay men's problem alone. It isn't only a problem for gay men and drug users, HIV affects everybody.

MARIANNE

Marianne, age twenty-six, has a university degree and is working as a professional for an international company. She tested positive two years ago and estimates that she acquired the virus at least five years ago.

IT ALL STARTED four years ago when my boyfriend told me just as we were in the process of splitting up. I was going in a different direction and felt that he was not the right guy for me, as much because I was keen on having babies and he wasn't showing any signs of being interested. He went for the test without telling me anything about it. One evening we were out and I kept talking about how much I wanted babies, when he suddenly burst out, telling me I would never have them. I didn't understand what was going on, and asked him why on earth he was saying that.

I suppose at the back of my mind there was some sort of awareness that we both had a chance of being positive because although I had never injected drugs, he had, and we had never used safer sex. It was a subject which we ignored, but suddenly I realized it could be real for both of us. I think we never talked about it before because we didn't want to know - sometimes you think it makes life easier not to know something rather than having to deal with it. However, when I asked him about AIDS, he kept on denying it and saying no, it wasn't that. Finally I came out and asked him if he'd had the test and he said, 'Okay, I did go and it's positive.'

I stopped trying to split up with him, and we started going

out again regularly because I wanted to support him; his positive status brought us together again. And of course there was the now the possibility that I was positive. But for me, it was much more that we had already been together for five years and that I went into a stage of total denial about myself, after finding out he was positive. I thought I might be lucky, I was in a schizophrenic state because I didn't know what to believe and I was too scared to go for a test and find out the truth. It was easier to deny it. However, after a year and a half we split up again for good and I started to date someone else. It was in this new situation that I realized I had to know, so finally I went for the test.

Going for the test wasn't at all straightforward. I was completely helpless. I rang up a friend whose father worked in the medical field and told him what was happening. He was the only friend I told and thankfully he organized the test for me, because I was paralysed and couldn't pick up the phone and say the words. A huge cloud of fears and insecurities hung over me.

The doctor I saw kept on telling me not to worry, I was probably negative. Certainly, except for my fears, I felt and looked the picture of health, but it's amazing to think now that a doctor would make that kind of judgement on how you looked. He took blood and I had to wait a week to get the result. It was tight timing because I was planning to spend the weekend with my new boyfriend and had decided I must know one way or the other before. When I went for the result the doctor wasn't on duty but he came in to tell me. We both arrived at the clinic together and when he saw me he said nothing except that I was to follow him in. Then he walked in front of me, getting into his profession, pulling on his white coat before he spoke to me. It was completely useless because it didn't make things better.

Even though I knew there was a chance I would be positive, I was devastated and almost completely ignorant about AIDS. The first thing that came to my mind was that I'd never have a relationship, never have children. What the fuck should I do with my life? Even though I was quite young, I'd always thought I'd have a family one day and then all of a sudden that possibility seemed to disappear. It's like your arm is getting cut off. I was so scared about AIDS before my diagnosis that I used to ignore articles in the media about it. I had the idea that people would assume I was positive if they saw me reading a book or article about the subject.

I went to see my new boyfriend knowing I would have to tell him. I had already told him that my ex-boyfriend was a drug user but I think he ignored the information. I worked for a bank at the time and what he saw was a young career girl he couldn't associate with something like HIV. So he was terribly shocked when I told him. We had made love already without condoms. It's one of those things you can be quite stupid about - but there are always two people being stupid, thinking I'll be one of the lucky ones who is negative. It hit me hard that I could not do that again, and after that I always insisted on using condoms. He went for a test which was negative, and I was so relieved. On top of all the feelings about being positive myself, it would have been much worse to know I'd given it to someone else.

That boyfriend dumped me soon afterwards. I think I understand. He was from such a different background, very conservative and settled. He led a really straight life and had never come in contact with anything like drugs. Once when were talking about HIV before I had the test, he told me his stepbrother was gay and that he was sorry for him because he had to live with the constant fear of becoming HIV positive. The next thing he knows is that I'm telling him that I am HIV positive, he slept with me, and really, he wasn't in such a different position from his stepbrother.

I think he really did like me, but he was in a complete state of shock and ultimately couldn't deal with it. The way he broke off with me hurt much more that the fact that we were splitting up. At first, after the break, he insisted that we stay friends, but after a while he didn't have the guts to face me and tell me he couldn't handle that any more. The last time I talked to him he said he would give me a ring another time but he never did. I am more angry that he couldn't face saying that's how it is, so instead he ran off like a child.

I never felt angry with my ex-lover. He was my biggest love and even if someone had been able to look into my future and tell me I would get infected from him, I probably wouldn't have done anything differently. I was very much in love with him, thought I couldn't live without him. Maybe I do believe in some kind of fate, or a predetermined life.

At the time I took the test we had been apart for a while and I had a new boyfriend so I didn't talk to him right away. Then, when we did talk he assumed I was positive before I told him and because he was bitter that I'd broken off our relationship he used that assumption to attack me. He told me I shouldn't have a relationship with anyone else. How could I bear to be responsible for someone else's death? For a long while all he wanted to do was hurt me because he had been so hurt himself.

We are in contact now; he's living in Hamburg and I'm in London. It's difficult because we have old friends in Hamburg and if you admit to being HIV positive it's like committing social suicide. You have to deal with other people's fears. It's strange, because I know a lot of people there who are all probably HIV positive, but it's never been an open subject.

You worry about telling even one person. Confidentiality is difficult to ask for - it might work with some people but usually you tell one person in confidence and that person tells someone, confidentially of course, and so it gets spread around. Everyone thinks they're terribly confidential because they've only told their closest friend! But eventually everyone knows including people you'd rather didn't. I try not to tell anyone at all. Even here in England, I keep two distinct sets of friends. I have one group I met through Positively Women, and another I've met through work, and I keep them totally apart. Of course it would be better if I didn't have to compartmentalize my life so rigidly, but only if things were completely different. Then it would be like telling someone you have cancer, which even if it's scary, is an accepted disease and you don't have to deal with the fearsome cloud people have about HIV. Usually very few people have good information or attitudes towards AIDS. Most simply ignore it, so once you tell them they have to take that on, plus all their own baggage. There are some people who either feel sorry for you or are overly friendly. I don't want that pity because in a peculiar sense it's quite tempting. If people feel sorry for you it would be easy to use it to your advantage, like getting everyone to do what you want simply because you are HIV positive. On the other hand there are people who are checking you out for being positive and making assumptions without ever really knowing you. I'm Marianne, I'm HIV positive, that's part of me but not everything.

I had been living in England off and on when I got my diagnosis in Germany. After, I returned to England. I didn't tell my family because my mother had recently discovered she had a brain tumour and my father was very ill and lost his job - it was a year when everything came at the same time and I couldn't bother them with yet another problem. I wasn't ready for it. Anyway I was living in London and that would probably have set up even more worries for them. Was I still all right? Did I have to go to hospital? Strangely, my mother once rang me in the morning, really upset because she had a dream that I had called her, moaning in pain, and in the dream she asked me if there was an emergency doctor I could ring in London. That made me shiver and I was about to say, 'You're right there is a lot wrong, but I'm not ill, not in pain.' It was as if she sensed something and it came out in a dream.

My parents are really average. Sometimes my mother tells me to be careful not to catch AIDS. One time I talked to her about a girlfriend who died of AIDS and that gave me a chance to touch on the subject. She was open about it but I still can't tell them. I left home when I was eighteen. I was angry with my parents at that time. I was the odd one out in the family and I believed they didn't understand me. I started to go out with boys early which my sisters didn't. My two sisters are very active in the church and their social lives revolve around the church. Thankfully my relationship with my parents is much better now.

There is no certainty about transmission of HIV. No one can predict 100 per cent who will be infected. The girlfriend of mine who died recently had a boyfriend for eight years who tested negative although they never used condoms. He must have been exposed to the virus. At Positively Women there are a number of women whose partners are negative. Obviously you either contract the virus through dirty needles or through sex, but you can't necessarily pin-point the exact day when it happened. In the end it doesn't matter because you have to deal with it and you can't change that. It doesn't help to go mad thinking about why you made the major mistake of sleeping with the wrong guy, or sleeping with someone at the wrong time in the wrong way.

For lots of people safer sex is a joke, it doesn't work. Everyone knows on one level that the virus is there, but hardly anyone uses condoms. Often people who are at an age where they are most 'at risk' are the ones who are unsettled or insecure. Having a relationship with someone is a delicate thing. If you meet someone and say, let's use condoms, you're afraid they might think you're the one who is positive and because of the stigma, who wants that? The stigma has got to go in order for people to admit to themselves that they might be at risk.

As far as I can tell, for men the ultimate sex is fucking. We tend to think it's the natural way of things - the woman can more easily get an orgasm by playing around, whereas the man has a sex drive attached to his penis. They need to have intercourse, or maybe they just think they need it. But once you're in bed with someone, it's difficult to draw a line because mostly it just happens, especially if you're not planning it in the first place. If you're even a bit drunk it's so easy to get carried away and ignore what the information says you should do. Once you're positive your attitude has to change, but there a plenty of untested people who may be positive, taking a gamble and persuading themselves they'll be lucky. Also a lot of heterosexuals don't know anyone who is positive, or at least they think they don't: it's something you read about in the newspaper. If the climate changed, allowing more people to come out and say 'I'm positive, I'm living with it, it's not the end of life', things might change. Then everyone could talk normally, without embarrassment. Now HIV and AIDS are embarrassing because of the negative images and associations which are attached to them, and they're frightening. A lot of people don't realize that there are many healthy people who are HIV positive. There's so much attached to it like death and suffering.

My generation, people between the ages of twenty-five and thirty, all grew up with the idea of free sex. When I started to have sex it was just a thing you did and it didn't really matter if you'd just met the guy in a club. You could go off, have sex, and never see each other again. All of a sudden AIDS appeared and made it necessary to rethink that attitude. Of course for women, birth-control has always been an issue, but even with that, if anything goes wrong you have the choice of an abortion. With HIV you can't sort anything out afterwards. I don't think the birth-control issue is closely connected with the HIV issue. Even if it's only a fantasy, the idea of having a baby can be quite romantic. On the other hand, a lot of women have rejected the Pill these days, so in a way it is an easy way to justify using a condom. You can get around the subject of HIV and AIDS by insisting on it for birth-control. Besides, if the guy doesn't understand that, he's an arsehole and should be dropped straightaway.

I think many women and men don't know how to use a condom and instead of making it a part of sex they may have an attitude which makes it impossible to use one without destroying the pleasure of fucking. If women put condoms on their lovers it would take the embarrassment out of the situation. Obviously if you are lying with someone about to have sex and then one of you has to get the condom from the bathroom, by the time it's on, the interest may have gone. It's true too that a lot of guys aren't very experienced in getting a condom on. I think both men and women should practice - women can do that by using a banana as a substitute. With experience (practise with the fruit) you can put one on the real thing with your mouth which for a guy is a pleasant experience, although sometimes they don't realize you're doing it. You have to be careful not to scratch the condom with your teeth. You just cover your teeth with your lips and push the condom down - it takes some practice but it's possible. It's part of sex. Men can get used to it and in a way it's quite exciting.

To tell you the truth, I haven't had sex with anyone for ages. I went through a very difficult period where I was confused about everything. After the split with my boyfriend, out of frustration I started to eat like a maniac. It was a way of treating myself and I put on a lot of weight. I was insecure, and it was only through getting to terms with being HIV positive that I've been able to deal with my own fears and my own personality. Now I actually feel stronger than I was before. I've started going out with boys again but not with anyone I really fancy - maybe I'm not ready yet. In your mind, you go through how you would tell someone, what would their reaction be? Or sometimes you meet a good guy and play with the thought of telling him. But I'm at the stage where it seems easier to be on my own.

In the beginning I went through a phase of thinking I could never have another relationship because who would go out with someone who was HIV positive? After I started to go to Positively Women I met a lot more women who were in the same situation and I saw that many of them were in normal relationships. I realized that it was a possibility but I still thought I couldn't handle worrying about someone else. If you're in love with someone you want the best for them and I felt I would rather protect the other person from any possible trauma. I'm getting more egotistic about it recently and think it might not be the best thing to go around defensively protecting someone else - everyone has to make decisions for themselves.

I'm quite sure I'll have a baby at some point. Maybe it won't happen and maybe it's part of the reason for not finding the right boyfriend. But I'm sure it's possible even if you're HIV positive. Some people blame an HIV positive woman for deciding to go ahead with a pregnancy and a lot of doctors will probably tell you it's better to have an abortion or never get pregnant. On the other hand, for other groups of women, it's probably as high or even higher a risk to have a child. For instance the risk of having a Downs Syndrome baby is probably more for a certain group of women, than for an HIV positive woman to have a positive baby. It's unfair, because instead of encouraging counselling, or even supporting a woman in her decision, doctors are negative and moralistic. There is still so much wrong information around about pregnancy and HIV. The worst are the GPs who think it's their duty to persuade women to have abortions. Often they give misinformation - you would think they should know the latest information and if they don't, admit it and get it.

I try to live a healthy life - except for smoking too much! I buy organic food, try not to abuse myself and even cut down on chocolate. But I'm not a fanatic about it. I went along to some macrobiotic cooking classes but it seemed too much to take on because either you do it properly or you don't do it at all. It would mean changing your whole lifestyle and I think, for myself, is it worth it? It would put stress on me and take some pleasure out of life. The best thing is to try to be happy, to enjoy yourself, and to find out what you enjoy and where you can get the pleasure. Since being HIV positive, I'm more self-centred. Not, I hope, in a way that hurts other people but I understand and take account of my own needs.

It's your mind which determines your life, whatever is in your mind is going to influence what happens. If you decide to die, you may very well die. It's possible to gain energy for life through being HIV positive too. I realize that much worse things can't come up, so I'm prepared to deal with everything. I am relaxed about things which other people get annoyed with; material things don't have as much meaning to me as they used to. Before if I messed up a new piece of clothing, it might have ruined my day but now it's unimportant. I have changed almost 100 per cent in my attitude to life.

There is a whole range of holistic therapies which can be useful, like meditation and visualization. In order to achieve a positive attitude, I try to keep my mind relaxed and I have found my own pattern of thinking which gives me support. Everyone has to find out for themselves what does them good or what they enjoy doing. Too much hard work at it leads to stress which is the opposite of what you need. Of course I'm scared of suffering from horrible diseases, but you don't necessarily have to get them. Sometimes I do think about moving somewhere else, to a seaside town, for instance, instead of working hard. Sometimes I think, what's the point of putting so much time into a career you might not enjoy the rewards of? But mainly I'm the type of person who carries on with life.

Thinking about death, fears of dying, are not necessarily anything to do with being HIV positive. Everyone has to die and no one knows exactly when they are going to, even if they're HIV positive. The only difference is that you grow up assuming you've been given eighty years of a life which will go through a number of stages. Suddenly someone like me knows there's a chance my life will stop before it should. But again this possibility isn't specific only to HIV infection.

Adopting a positive attitude towards life would do people in general good. Too many people are negative towards life and death. Death is unknown and you don't know what might happen afterwards. But there are cultures which celebrate death instead of mourning, whereas in our western cultures we are frightened and think it's something to cry about.

On the way to my girlfriend's funeral I carried a lovely flower arrangement which was obviously for a funeral. On the train I could see other people were staring at me and I could see them wondering who had died, what was my connection to the dead person? I had dressed like I would to go and meet her, not in a sombre suit, so it was clear I wasn't a relative. After arriving at the station, one man actually came up to me and asked who it was who'd died. Maybe there is also something about mortality which some people are oddly attracted to because it touches them in a strange way and brings life back to its essentials. It is a dramatic moment. People are left behind.

I realized through the illness of my girlfriend that the thing I hate most is when other people get a sorrowed voice when they talk to you. I have adopted such a different attitude towards death and I now imagine it much more like a big party where you get to meet everyone you ever cared about before who is already dead. You lose your body but you join a big crowd of dead souls.

When I was first diagnosed, it was on my mind all the time, it was the first thing I thought about when I woke up. I'd sit in tea-breaks thinking that no one knew about it and who else might be positive? I tested my glands at least twenty times a day, so much so that all that pressing gave me swollen glands one time! I didn't think I wanted to go anywhere for support. I had awkward ideas about it: it would be hippie-ish, people would sit around a table drinking tea and moaning about their lives. But in fact I eventually realized I needed to talk to others in my position. The friend who organized the test for me found out about the Terrence Higgins Trust. I went there to get counselling which wasn't totally satisfying because my English wasn't great and when I asked about diseases I could get and other information, I wasn't familiar with all the words she used. She told me to get a dictionary which wasn't very sensitive.

I had already looked up Positively Women in the phone book so I decided to give counselling another chance. Later on the same day I went to one of their support groups which I really enjoyed. I was surprised at the mixture of women. I could identify with their lifestyles and their attitudes to life. I realized you could be positive, happy, and you didn't have to sit at home and think about dying. I enjoyed it because it also gave me the opportunity to talk frankly about my life which is something I usually don't do, even with my closest friend. I go to a certain point but then stop because I want to protect myself, so I censor the information I give out. It's not only factual information, but what my worries are, what I feel, what my nightmares are. If you talk about everything you give a certain power to the person who hears you. Once you've said it, you can't take it back. You never know how long a friendship will last and you're afraid of what might be used against you.

Perhaps I have a negative attitude towards friends, but I know I've had close relationships and all of a sudden they've changed, you're more like strangers than friends. If you are in a support group, you're not necessarily close to anyone and you trust that everything said will stay in the room; you believe that because you're all in the same situation.

At the moment I don't feel I need support. HIV is not a big issue in my life; I hardly think about it. Occasionally I go to a support group but it's mainly to see the other women again. It can feel awkward because you go through different stages and if a new woman is there you can recognize and relate to what she's going through but you relate to it as a part of your past.

I admire people who work for organizations like Positively Women. To work there as a volunteer gave me a good insight into how difficult it can be. You have to like people a lot, while understanding that you're not going to be able to relate to every woman, her life, or her personality, equally. You have to put your own feelings aside and be there to help. It's a lot of power, or, perhaps a better word is energy. I know I would be tempted to shake some people and tell them they're getting on my nerves, talking rubbish. Everyone, HIV positive or not, has a different personality. And in Positively Women you meet such different people. No one can expect to get on with everyone but if you are working there you have to keep to a professional plane, at the same time that you're touched on a personal level. You're having to deal with private, personal parts of women's lives. Sometimes it's not being HIV positive which is hopeless for a woman, it's her whole life which is in a mess. Then it's hard to know where to start or how to sort it out. I found that difficult. You have to have the gift of being a good social worker and I'm an aggressive person in a way, so I don't think I had that gift.

It's important Positively Women exists and not only because more and more women are being diagnosed. Many women need or want a women's group for support. Women who are HIV positive want to talk about their lives, about babies, and relationships among many other things, in their own way. Because being gay is also stigmatized, gay men already have an experience of dealing with a difficult challenge, with something which changes their lives from the assumed heterosexual path, and which changes their relationship to people. When this disease showed itself among gay men they had the possibility of falling back on an existing network. Gay men used their already existing scene to deal with the disease and sometimes if you go to an AIDS organization it will be 99 per cent gay men. It can be an awkward feeling for a woman, although I don't think it's intentional at all. But sometimes you feel a bit left out, you don't know anyone and it appears cliquy.

Women have more problems getting organized but it's not that they're incapable of it. It's much more to do with women's lifestyles. A lot of positive women have children so it's difficult to take on something else. I stopped going to Positively Women when I didn't have the time for it. I imagine that in a couple of years time if I give up working and have a baby, I'll be more flexible about my time, and maybe I'll go back and do some voluntary work. Now I don't need the group and I don't have the time, but if I hadn't found Positively Women in the first place I might not be able to say that today.

MAGGIE

*Maggie is thirty-six years old and has a
nine-year-old son. She lives in a council
flat in London and has worked for
Positively Women since the spring of
1991. She has been HIV antibody positive
for four years.*

I WAS BORN in Canada in 1956 after my parents emigrated
there from Ireland with my two older brothers. When I was
two my mother left, taking us back to Ireland with her. She
was an independent woman who moved around and stayed away
from her family. We were brought up as Catholics although I
was never sent to a convent school.

Our mother always told us that if anyone asked about our
father, we should say that he was working abroad. We all felt
a certain amount of insecurity about our situation. Then one
day when I was about five the absent father turned up, out of
the blue, on the doorstep. My brothers recognized him right
away but I didn't know who he was. Someone had to say, 'That's
your father just walked in, come to Ireland to see you.' He
spent the day with us and we all had a great time. Later, when
my mother came home from work, it was obvious she wasn't
expecting him. He stayed the night, sleeping in a room on his
own, and then the next day he left and from there he disappeared. He must have got some money from somewhere, and
that was it, he got a boat out of Ireland and he's never been
seen or heard of since.

We hadn't expected to see him when he showed up and it
must have affected my mother. I heard tales that their differences
were over religion, that he didn't like all the Catholic stuff. I

also heard that he liked to gamble which my mother wasn't prepared to put up with. All through my childhood she never spoke about him at all, which seems fair enough to me.

Everything I now know came from my grandmother after my mother died. Their relationship was just one of those family secrets, an unmentionable topic I never even thought to ask about while my mother was alive. After she died I started having silly little fantasies about him, and it was only after I had my son that I realized what my mother must have gone through, all on her own with three children. That stopped the fantasies. He could have sent her some money. Apparently at the beginning he sent little bits, but that soon stopped.

My mother stayed on her own until she died, but she managed to stay lively and active, and she always had a boyfriend. Because she lived on her own with three children, she had complete control of her finances; she had no man to account to, or a man out of work to worry about - she had none of that pressure. She had a boyfriend who would come and visit her every evening and always leave by eleven o'clock. At the weekends he would stay, sleeping in a separate room. She worked at the school canteen and with old people and was always involved in the community. She enjoyed herself. Even though she never lived with anyone else, I know she intended to. Before she got cancer, she was planning to get a divorce, which for a Catholic is a big thing. She waited until all her children were more or less grown up and then she said, 'Look, it's like this, if you don't mind I want to get divorced, and I want to marry David, and we're going to emigrate to Australia.' But then she got cancer and died and she couldn't do any of it.

I was really close to my father's side of the family, particularly my grandmother and grandfather. He was a bit of a nut case, in fact all his family, the great-uncles, were a bit nutty. There was child abuse in my Catholic family: old men with their granddaughters and great-nieces. It was never common knowledge or at least no adults ever talked about it. One of the great-uncles abused me. My aunt found out what happened and she said, 'Okay, you don't ever have to go down there again.' She never told my mother, but she stopped it and I think she did it in the right way. The only problem was that nobody ever talked to me about it; it wasn't until I was seventeen and living in London that I mentioned it to anyone, and not until I was twenty-eight and had my son that I ever talked about the fact that I was sexually abused as a child and that there were all these undercurrents going on in my supposedly so Catholic, proper family.

I didn't know what happened to me was abuse. I knew something was wrong but I blamed myself totally for letting it happen. When you grow up Catholic you have a guilt thing all the time, you go to confession and you think, my god, did I let that happen? I would like to talk to an analyst about what happened to me because there are still things I want to clear up about it, but I only want to talk in depth to somebody who doesn't know me. That would be the only way I could explore the experience fully.

One of my brothers emigrated when he was seventeen and that was very sad. Nobody ever talked about his leaving, I suffered it in silence with such heartbreak. Then my eldest brother who became my guardian at age twenty-one after my mother died, left for London and I followed suit. He suggested I come because there was nothing in Northern Ireland for us. It was true. We were Catholics and we lived in a Protestant town. There was no life there for us and it was especially difficult for people our age.

When I arrived in London it was terrible. I had never drunk before, but in London I got into alcohol and cigarettes and all sorts of other drugs which were going around because at least they made me feel good for a while. For a few years everything was unbearable, almost suicidal. I felt as if nobody loved me: my brother had a girlfriend, everybody had somebody, but I was alone. As a child, my mother had protected me. She was a strong mother, and quite a dominant woman. After she died, I thought I was free and could do as I pleased. I may have had the freedom but in reality I was insecure and unprepared for life in a strange city.

My mother had been ill off and on for a long time - over the years she'd been in hospital with various complaints but they weren't life threatening. The cancer got her within six months; she went straight downhill. I didn't realize she was going to die until the day my brother took me aside and told me our mother was never going to come out of the hospital, she was not going to survive. That evening she died. I didn't even know she had cancer; I could see she was getting thinner and thinner but I thought as nobody said anything, obviously she was going to get well again. At the time, I was still a Catholic and I'd pray, worried that she was in such a state, even thinking sometimes that it would be better if she died. But I didn't really believe for a moment that it would happen.

I have definitely avoided talking about death with my son. I keep assuming that if I get ill, it will be a gradual thing. I can't picture getting ill like my mother and dying so quickly. If I had to go into the hospital and they told me something really serious was happening, like PCP, that would be the time to talk to him. But I realize that he should be prepared and that maybe it is a good idea to introduce him to the idea when I'm really well. He will have had years of me being well, but if he's prepared and I do get ill there will be no shock. He would be able to understand that someone can have the HIV virus, continue to be well for ages and maybe get ill later on but recover. Within that context he might be able to understand that there is a chance you could die from it in the end. When I look at it that way, I think I really do have to talk to him. But it's still one of those things I can't bring myself to do and I don't believe I will be able to without help.

I haven't told any of my family, including my two brothers, that I'm HIV positive. They should know, mainly because of my son as he might need them someday. But again, rationally I know I should do it, but emotionally I haven't been able to accomplish it yet.

During my first few years in London I tried cutting my wrists, I took sleeping tablets, and I drank too much - it was clearly a cry for help, wasn't it? Finally I met Tim who was a really nice man. He was very kind and we had a very stable relationship for about seven years. His family, particularly his mother who lived in Suffolk, provided me with much needed security. Tim and I were good friends as well, the sort who had a lot of fun together. But it wasn't meant to last. I left him about ten years ago, at which point I went off the rails again for a while.

Then I met my son's dad, R. We met through friends and I thought, he's fine, he'll do, a nice secure man - all this even though I knew he'd been using drugs. By then my ideal was to stop work, find a secure flat and get pregnant. But as soon as I got pregnant, I didn't want to be with him any more - it was a mistake and our personalities weren't suited at all. We ended up staying together for a couple of years, until the baby was two, and then I got him out. Separating from him was difficult - eventually he left probably because I was so horrible and nasty to him that he couldn't take it any more.

Well before he left he'd got back into drugs, using heroin and that's when I started using them too. It was as if eighteen months of life completely disappeared. I wasn't into drugs when I had my son. That happened later. He was so tiny when he was born I couldn't believe it. When I look at later photographs, there is my son's father, totally out of his head, and there I am, a washed out mother, and there is this big chubby baby. Separating from R took me away from the heroin. It put a big gap there immediately because nobody was bringing it in to the flat and that made it easy to stop. However, I was depressed and I wasn't coping with anything. So a while later I got back on drugs all by myself.

I met John through a friend. He didn't take heavy drugs although he'd have some at parties and liked to go to the pub to have a drink. I liked his personality and I suppose, typically for me, I looked at him and saw a practical man who could offer me security. We were seeing each other for a year before it came out that there was a possibility that he could be HIV positive. Mind you, I probably had the same possibilities myself because I'd been with R, although the thought never entered my mind at the time. John decided to take the test and found out he was positive. I assume I got the virus from him. I remember getting ill within a few weeks of getting together with him which had never happened to me while I was with R. I've seen R in the street and if he had the virus, I reckon he'd be ill by now, which he's not, because he abuses himself so much. The last time I slept with him was six months before my son was born; he's nine now so that was a long time ago. John had spent time in Africa and knowing what he was up to, I guess the chances are it was him.

After he found out he was positive, I went for a test. It too was positive. We had been on the verge of breaking up before all this happened but we stayed together for a while longer, for moral support really. I ended up feeling sorry for him even though by that time I disliked him intensely.

Eventually it was clear that it was no good and that I couldn't go on feeling guilty about him. By then I didn't care if I was on my own for the rest of my life. I found out I was positive about five years ago. Soon after I was on my own with a five year old kid. Your mind can get really good at blocking things out and I have to dig around to find memories about exactly what happened. I had been going to psychotherapy before my HIV diagnosis because of the relationship with John. I couldn't cope, my reactions to him were really extreme and I'd burst into tears all the time. I thought there were definite problems coming up and that they must have to do with the abuse I'd been through as a child. I got to the psychotherapy unit at St Thomas' hospital and the therapist said: 'Well my dear, what's your problem?' And I said, 'Oh, I don't know, blah-blah-blah, I was abused as a child, I can't seem to keep a relationship together, I'm a very jealous person, will you help me?' 'Well', he said, 'really, you're a big woman now, you should have dealt with the child abuse by this point. And about your relationship - people do play games with each other, maybe this man's playing a game, and why don't you get rid of him?' More or less, that's what he said.

Then I blurted out, 'Well really, all that's immaterial because I've recently found out that I'm HIV positive and I think that's probably my biggest problem at the moment.' He replied, 'Fine, okay, that's really the icing on the cake as far as your life is concerned. We'll give you therapy for four months and you'll be as right as rain.' And it's true, it worked. I had one-to-one sessions with him once a week and he changed the way I thought. I learned to take the pressures off myself and not to put them on other people. It helped me with my son; I was having a hard time being a mother and I wasn't coping with the rest of my life either. I would get upset when he went into a tantrum. I'd start thinking of all the pressure I put on him to be a perfect child and to behave himself, as well as putting it on myself to be a perfect mother, to have a perfect child. It was as if I was saying he shouldn't be having tantrums or I should be able to talk him out of them.

To start off with the therapy took the word 'should' out. We all make mistakes, none of us are perfect, none of our children are perfect. Every time I find myself not coping I think, okay, what's really going on here? I repeat to myself that I do worthwhile things in my life; I have much more realistic expectations from life now.

Around the time you first get diagnosed positive, you're bursting to tell people. I told the wrong person, when he was very drunk he told his girlfriend and she, in turn, told other people. John didn't want anyone to know and he was very angry that I'd let the news out. In therapy I was able to ease my guilt by realizing that we all make mistakes and that happened to be a really delicate one, but there was nothing I could do about it after it happened. Even after we split up I wasn't supposed to tell anyone because of him. I don't think women are as secretive about being HIV positive because women can sit and

71

really talk to each other and most men can't do that - they never learned how to talk intimately to male friends.

Through all the time of finding out and doing therapy I took courses. I was doing O-level English when I found out I was HIV positive and continuing with the class every week was one of the ways I kept sane. My class had the most ordinary people in it and there I was with the most extraordinary emotional stuff going on in my head. It was therapeutic to bring up the subject of AIDS and HIV now and again and get people talking about it. Also I was doing an evening course in mime which I kept up for two years even though I wasn't very good at it. I liked it because it was physical and completely different from anything else in my life. It helped keep me together because I thought if I can keep doing such physical stuff, then I must be staying healthy.

I was obsessed with staying healthy. I smoked but wanted to stop. In the beginning a lot of the crying I did was over my son. I wondered what would happen to him if I died. What if I only had another five years? I decided that obviously I had to live as long as possible; every time I had a cigarette I'd think, oh god, I can't do this to him. I stopped smoking more or less, although I still have the odd one. I kept drinking though. At the time I suppose I thought that if I stopped smoking that was a big step and enough for the time being. I got into vitamins and all the different things which at the time you were advised might be good to take. It was also the start of all the different diets I've gone through: eating only raw food, eating only cooked food, eating only whole grain food and organic food, and not eating sugar. Now I'm trying to find one where you can mix it all up! If I drink, maybe all the healthy eating goes out the window but my whole life can't be a regime. Still, if I really want to see my son a grown-up man then I've got to do as much as I can to lengthen my life. If I didn't have him, I'm not sure what my attitude would be, I might think, fuck it, I'm going to enjoy myself. I go to bed early and try to get proper sleep. I've started doing T'ai C'hi and I'm thinking this could work, it might really do something for my white blood cells. There's always the search for something which will help.

There is no other family for my son to go to - there are no parents or grandparents, aunts or uncles, no one he is close to. We have a very close relationship but sometimes in the back of my head I try to distance myself from him a bit. I don't know if it's the right thing to do, but sometimes it occurs to me that I have pushed him off on other people almost as a way of getting him used to the possibility. Now he's at an age where he's choosing people he really likes to see and that feels good to me.

Sex. Hah! What about it? I call them interludes and I've had some. My first happened when I went on holiday and met an older man. He was a nice guy and really good with my son, and I was impressed. I told him what I been through and he was all right about it, so I slept with him, not getting too close. He always used condoms. That was a holiday romance. Since then I've had other little interludes in which I've been honest and up front about my HIV status, and so far I've never been rejected.

Sometimes people hide behind their fear of telling because they assume they'll be rejected. They decide it's easier not to put themselves in that situation. I believe it's not a healthy thing to hide and cut off from things completely. In the future you will come across men you are attracted to and when they find out you're positive, yes, they might walk out the door. What are you going to do then? If they do walk out it's just as well, because they're not worth knowing. There is also the possibility they won't walk out and you'll never know unless you overcome the fear of rejection.

When you're HIV positive and you're told you can't have any children or more of them, you feel terrible. It was another thing that made me feel different from all the other women I saw walking down the street and I definitely went through feeling an incredibly strong sense of being completely different from everyone else, and of been denied so much. Some time later they discovered I had pre-cancerous cells and I remember coming out of my GPs' surgery after listening to him trying to convince me that it wasn't anything serious. But for me, it was a huge thing. I burst into tears again and again - how could this be happening to me after all I'd been through? I don't know how I coped during that period. Perhaps you go into a state of shock and don't even realize it. When I found out I was positive, nobody said to me, Maggie, for the next six months or more, be very good to yourself. At the same time you experience all the shock and despair, you also hurry up and do all the things you wanted to do in your life. No more wasting time.

I'm working at Positively Women now and I want the job to go really well, I want to be really good at it and get involved in everything. Different things inspire me at different times, but I know that in the future I want to have an amazing adventure of some kind and to take my son with me. I want to travel and if I ever have enough money, what I'd love to do is go to Australia, into the outback. If it wasn't for HIV, I'd be thinking, okay for the next five years I'm going to save up and put money away and then go off and do it. Now I'm in a job where I can earn some decent money and I want to have that adventure with my son as soon as I can.

Sometimes I wonder, Why me? Why am I HIV positive? Because I'm really stupid? Did I lead my life in such a wrong way? The wrong places at the wrong times, doing the wrong things with the wrong people? Or is it fate? Here you are, this is what you've got to deal with. Maybe it's all complete chance. It's just a load of chaos out there and it depends where you were one day, or the next day, which bus you got on to. I can't see any predestined plan into which my life fits. Whatever the reason, or bad luck, I'm learning to accept myself as I am and to get on with living my life as best I can.

MAYA

Now twenty-one and out as a lesbian at university, Maya is at once enjoying the proximity of being with people her own age - while fully realizing the distance created by experience.

I

I WAS NEVER a very good junkie. It never gave me status or recognition. Maybe it gave me a fallacious sense of belonging. I never saw light or logic in what I did or who I was (am). What it gave me was retreat. The rush of gear shooting to my head is the most memorable experience I will ever have. I say this with certainty, for I find myself grappling with something physical, emotional, intellectual and sensorial - all in a gouached abstraction. There was a weekly trip up Charing Cross Road. Wandering in and out of shops to steal books. Reading, another retreat from the police, the social workers and Mr and Mrs Public. In fact, all otherness that conglomerates as the nebulous They. I was fifteen and kind of alone. Too much care, too much institutionalization. Chaotic years. Too ill, too frequently. Tolerance levels shooting all over the place. Heroin OD. Coma - Woke up to HIV. 1986.

II

INDIA, 1989
'I almost forgot Christmas had come and gone this year. It feels good. Received your letter today, about half an hour ago. It prompted me to write what I've been staving off these past few

75

weeks. Often felt caught between wanting to write (communicate?), yet stopping - to feel and smell the air here without reflecting back to England and all I've left behind. Wanting to keep the two separate. Not altogether possible. You've made London connect again.

'It's raining now... for the first time since I arrived. In the morning the city will be clean. On Christmas Eve we drove down through Fort William around dusk. Sounds of conches and crows. The light is so different here, then it fades - quickly.

'It was the best time to see this multi-tiered life. There stood the Victoria Memorial, soliloquizing on a glory that's long since spent. At the gates, the vendors and the shanties. Flies and stagnant water. Bare bulbs and naked children. Hinduism teaches them perseverance and tolerance. Atheists might claim it's an effective Explanation and means of silencing the poor. I don't quite think so. I never quite think so.

'My head is throbbing. Is there always something left to say? I am thinking about dignity. Here it slaps me in the face. How much we strive for dignity. Some semblance of control? Underneath I feel myself give way. My mind exposed and splattered for all of you to see. Me and my hammer. Skull cracks a little more. Gauging out eyes; out of mind, out of sanity. Every context is sense-LESS - if the past could be forsaken let this be a new time...

'It's that cracking feeling surging up. Sometimes it knocks on my head. I lock myself in and don't look out. Introversion? Maybe. I take my mind for a walk, "don't look back" - so I do; to hear that tapping all over again.'

III

1991
Fast approaching that quieter time of night again. Typing reminds me of dissertation - all androgynous and ink blots; dissertation - tapping reminder of exam results. *Newsnight* was

about Euthanasia. Recollections of conversations with S, with me and me and me again. Reasons, reasons, everybody needs reasons for something that in actual fact is nothing. Nothingness is as frequent as rain here. In more arid climates it's welcomed, prayed for through all that striving, thrusting and beaten by the elements.

Beaten, battered. Resilient.

Thoughts flow over me, around, about, everywhere. The rain keeps falling. Persistent intermittentness. That's just it.

Reflections on 'PARADISE'. People responded. To what? A canvas, an image, an Ideal? Back to androgynous again. N - trying to ward off another reality, another dimension. No freedom to think. No courage to think? But conceptual art is wholly too wholesome. That unrefined white. Granary. Grain, bits, lumps - texture. PULSE... reduced to singularity, completely. Absolutely.

At leisure I can smile about the will to live. Elan, minus the acute accent because I can't find the key. Left my notebook upstairs. Funny how V emptied recollections of last summer's writing. The exact same notions of thought and lucidity. Nuggets of truth wrapped in words of persuasion. Religion, like doctors, reducing truths to truisms. The night is trickling in. Wet and cool and cool and definite.

I still maintain, Nothing changes. Colours, which then evaporate. Trying to think some sense of the senseless. Can any strength come from so much doubt? Everything, perhaps, is musting. Thoughts jumping, no moving - hither and thither (like a slippery slimy rhyme!) and the original thought is difficultly retrieved. Like differentiating the empirical from the memorable.

I V

AUGUST 1991
Now I am laughing.
I see it like this,
A perfect sphere. I travel on the inside of that
sphere as an infinity of paths with a multiplicity
of experience. AIDS is one of these experiences,
but one that persistently taps then throbs
then taps inside me.
I am Necessarily strengthened by it.
It splashes the inside of that sphere with a
vitriolic crimson. My eyes are sore.
Trying always to remember the thought as it came.
But then went. As it always does.
Rhythmical, mimical sameness. This sameness is
never washed away by the rain, or lessened,
or dulled or obliterated.

OCTOBER 1991
And finally, how we thrive on nostalgia!
Memorabilia. KNOT
Not being tired. Not being ill. Not swallowing pills.
Of course, everything Else which is good and
positive and stimulating carries on;
with this tapping reminder.

DECEMBER 1991
Perhaps without the emergence of Positively Women I would
not have found the friendship, love and support that has allowed
me to become settled and feel acknowledged and cared for.

I suppose there are no real aspirations or hopes for the future - simply because here, today, is what's important.

KATE

Kate is thirty-one and has been diagnosed HIV positive since 1987. She works full-time for Positively Women and is an editor of this book.

IT'S HARD TO write about yourself, especially when you're not used to it and when most of the writing you've done till now has been something you don't enjoy, or more often hate: school work, exam papers, letters to people you've never seen, thanking or asking or complaining. For me, writing has always been something done in haste or under pressure with no particular thought or planning going into it and little, if any, pleasure or satisfaction derived from it. The idea of someone else reading what I've written fills me with dread, it leaves you vulnerable, open to ridicule and criticism. The shortcomings of the language available to us means you will probably be misunderstood anyway. Why did I ever agree to write this in the first place? I guess compiling this book seemed like a good idea at the time. Something important to do.

So where do I begin? How can I make sense out of the chaos? How can I impose structure on what defies structure? There's no beginning, middle and end - only a hotch-potch of memories which dim and fade at times, and at others seem to appear unexpectedly from nowhere I can recognize - perhaps from the smell of a match that has burned to the end or the after-taste of a particular dish. Memories which evolve and mutate so much that I'm no longer sure what really happened, or even if it happened at all.

Memories do even stranger things in families. These memories are not owned by one person but collectively, and they are rewritten, negotiated and used as ammunition and blackmail material in our power struggles. These warped memories of the past shape us, tell us who we are; they are used to blame, to create and sustain myths which bind and imprison and stop us from growing. In my family these myths have become so strong and constraining that we are like actors and actresses in a play whose script we know by heart but believe we cannot change. My part in this play is well-defined and there is little flexibility or room for negotiation. It is more about their needs and expectations than mine, although for me it is sometimes comforting and usually easier to conform to.

None of my family were surprised when I told them I was HIV positive. Sad perhaps. Supportive certainly. But not surprised. It was almost as if it were expected of me. I have always been their collective 'problem' and sometimes their collective 'cause'. Often a focus for their guilt, I have repre-sented all that is shameful, all that is secret and unsaid. So HIV fit the pattern nicely. It's still hard to get taken seriously by them, no matter what I do. Rocking the family boat is taboo. When faced with the options of change, reassessment and pro-gression or silence and denial the family closes ranks and unites in defence of the status quo. This safety is suffocation.

In the same way that the myths we create in families can limit our options and stop us from changing our behaviour, the myths surrounding AIDS also serve to keep people comfortable and secure and to maintain a distance and difference between themselves and those living with HIV. It's always someone else's problem. Societies can blame and create scapegoats and inno-cent victims and justify their lack of change in behaviour and complacency. Myths fast become accepted 'facts' and as such provide a rationale for the very real forms of prejudice, dis-crimination and oppression experienced by those of us with HIV.

This is why those of us who are able, in whatever way we can, must speak up, act up, and challenge these myths.

SILENCE = DEATH

I was conceived in Aden, a tiny place to the south of Saudi Arabia. I was born in West Sussex. My mother was a young middle-class woman working for the Foreign Office in the Middle East, my father, an Indian doctor also based there. I was the result of a brief affair and they broke off all contact with each other after she returned to England to have me. The family never spoke about my father. They still refuse to. My mother only told me about him when I was thirteen and has refused to speak of him since. I suppose that back in the 1960s having an illegitimate child was not the kind of thing nice middle-class girls did, or talked about, a lot. Especially if the child was not quite white. So perhaps I was set up as the 'black' sheep way back at the start!

It was 1961 and we lived with my grandparents. I was their first grandchild, doted on and spoiled rotten. My mother went to work as a secretary in a local rubber company and my grandmother took care of me during the day. Mum met my stepfather when I was about two and a half. He had recently left film school and wanted to be a writer; meanwhile he was caretaker of an empty factory owned by the company where my mother worked. They soon fell in love and got married and we went to live in South London with my new grandmother. Mum got pregnant with my brother and dad went to work for a publishers. As usual I got spoiled by an adoring grandmother. After a while we moved to our own place in West London and then my sister was born too. From the start I didn't like the new babies - I don't think it was jealousy but rather a lack of interest. I'm not a maternal person. Never have been and doubt I ever will be. Even back then I told my mother that if I ever got pregnant by mistake she would have to look after the child. The only time in my life I ever wanted a baby was when I was diagnosed HIV positive and told I could never have one. Once I felt that option had been taken away from me, I felt broody and envious of women who were mothers. But only for a week or so. And now I know that pregnancy is a real possibility women living with HIV there's no desire whatsoever. But at least I know that I have the choice.

My parents were quite a modern young 1960s couple and we always had writers and publishers, artists and film makers around the house. When they had parties I used to sit on the stairs, hidden from view to spy on them. Sometimes if I was lucky they'd let me come down and join them for a while. Then I started school which I hated. Especially the toilets which were horrible and dirty with that hard tracing paper instead of tissue and the boys would always come into the girls' ones and force the doors open while we were having a piss. Sometimes kids got their heads stuffed down the toilet bowls as well. So I mainly wet my knickers and got sent to the school nurse for dry ones and then had to stand at the back of the class for the rest of the day. If I wasn't standing at the back for that it would be because I wouldn't say my name when the teacher called the register. I never liked public speaking, which is ironic considering how much of it I have to do now. We had a running battle which neither of us ever won - the teacher because she never broke me - and me because I invariably landed up at the back with my hands on my head for hours on end. Quite often I missed all this conflict - in the afternoons when I had to sit all alone in the canteen staring at my untouched plate of cold stewed cabbage and swede and my inedible bowl of tapioca or cold, lumpy, puke-inducing pink custard. I liked these afternoons best. Not happy memories but the only ones I can find.

My best friend Rachel's parents and mine became friends and the two families started spending a lot of time together. Years later my mother told me that my dad and Rachel's mum were having an affair and used to leave the kids with her while they went off for the weekend. I never noticed. I thought we were all happy families.

My dad decided he wanted to write full-time and we moved down to Sussex. We spent the next seven years there till I was fourteen. I liked my life, I liked my schools, I liked my friends during this time. In the late 1960s or early 1970s my dad started teaching film studies at the British campus of an American college near to where we lived. My mother also started working there and from that time on we were always surrounded by students - in our home, in their homes, at the college.

This was when I first came into contact with illegal drugs. Drugs were what the older people whom I admired took; they went with the kind of music I was listening to; they were about being creative and cool. My doctor prescribed me valium for insomnia and I tried mixing it with cider at parties. I had the occasional puff on a joint. It made me feel grown-up. When I was thirteen we found out that my dad was having an affair with one of his female students. She was a family friend whom I had loved and trusted, and I felt let down and confused and really fucking furious as hell. My mum told me, then she told me about my real father, then she told me about my dad and my friend Rachel's mother and how their marriage had been on the rocks for a long time. All in the space of about five minutes. I was devastated. I knew they argued but I'd thought this was normal. I always believed my parents were not like other people's, that they were special, more together, wiser. As I lay in my room digesting and trying to make sense of this revelation all of a sudden I felt much older. The sense of bitterness, betrayal and anger was of an intensity I have never allowed my self to feel since. Perhaps your mind builds in automatic defence mechanisms. Perhaps you are immunized for life. I listened to my records and wept for the loss of my innocence and for the end of my parent's marriage. For the end of my childhood. I wept for hours and hours until drained of emotion I felt good, stronger. More in control.

I didn't find that safe emotional void again until I tried heroin. It all seems too corny now but that was how it seemed at the time. I guess self-indulgent amateur dramatics in times of stress have always been my forte.

My dad got a job teaching in the States. A chance for us all to start afresh. We set off for our new life on a Polish ship from Tilbury. The grim train ride there through a grey and dismal city, East London at it's worst, reinforced my desire to get away both physically and mentally as far and as fast as possible. So like many before me I approached America with renewed hope and excitement and a vision of the country learned from the TV. It began badly - I was seasick to the point of seriously considering putting an end to my misery by jumping ship mid Atlantic - but it ended worse than I could have imagined.

Arriving in rural New Hampshire was comparable to being dumped in Twin Peaks on a bad day. The afternoon we arrived in our new house, a large and typically New England place on the edge of a stunningly beautiful lake, a teenage girl and her friend appeared at the front door. She was covered with blood, her head smashed open, and fresh blood continued to pour onto the floor where she stood. An accident in the woods. A few days later we discovered the previous family who had lived in the house had lost their daughter when she drowned in the lake while playing with local kids. The man down the road had just shot his son, mistaking him for a deer in the woods. Everyone had a gun lying around on the kitchen table or next to the bed. Everyone drank and took as many drugs as they could afford or steal. The population was, and no doubt still is, made up of the weirdest and most fucked up individuals I've ever encountered. Incest, murder or shooting accidents, arson, drugs and arms running were all to rural New Hampshire what jumble sales and church socials are to rural England. Basically, as the locals used to say, you either got out of it or you got out. And as the second option was not open to me, I took the first.

Within a couple of weeks we all started school. My dad started teaching and moved in with one of his students (now my stepmother, Lucy) in another town. And so the great new life began. At the high school I was attending there were, like in teenage films, two basic tribes of pupils. Firstly the 'nice' ones who worked diligently to get good grades: the girls wore twin sets and pearl earrings; the boys dressed smart and had short hair. They drove cars to school once they were sixteen. They never got caught smoking outside, didn't do drugs and were virgins. Then there were the rest of us: the only cars we drove to school were stolen; we wore Levis and Indian shirts and the boys had long hair too. We got caught smoking joints in the toilets and at any time a large percentage of us would be suspended from school. Although school work was no problem for me, my A grades were often reduced to Cs because of my extra-curriculum activities. One time I was suspended for two weeks because a friend spiked my drink with LSD at a school dance. I'd never done acid before. The police took me home while I threw up in the back of their car, and after they'd strip-searched me I was forced under the shower to wash off the vomit. The next day they drove back to make me look at and smell the damage. After that not a week went by without them hassling me and accusing me (wrongfully, most of the time) of doing one thing or another.

By this time my mother was in a serious state. Dumped on her own, forty miles from the nearest town, with three kids, one of whom was fast becoming a mother's nightmare of a teenage monster, and with no close friends to turn to, she not surprisingly cracked up. By the time winter came things turned worse and the six foot snow drifts, situated permanently outside the door, reinforced in a physical way the isolation she was experiencing in her head. By the beginning of December my mother weighed five and a half stone. I used to come home at night sometimes and find her wandering around lost in the snow, dressed only in a nightdress, out of her head on valium. At times she became like a small child crying out for someone to take care of her. It was from this time onwards that I started feeling responsible for her, so in a way gained power over her. I was, however, in no great state myself to take charge. Fucked up by the upheaval in my life, beginning to be fucked up by the drugs and certainly by the alcohol, fucked up by other people's perceptions of who I was and by the realization that my parents were not gods but fragile and fallible human beings,

I was ill-prepared for, or able to cope with, the new responsi-
bilities I now faced.

The hardest thing for me was that I was expected to keep
all this a secret. Especially from my brother and sister. I was
told they were too young to know or understand what was really
going on. It's hard to believe they didn't pick up on all the
stressful and strange vibes being hurled around, but years later
I asked them about it and they insist they were blissfully unaware of it all.

Christmas was the worst. My paternal grandmother came
over to visit from England. Dad moved back in with us for
the duration of the stay and we had to work even harder on the
pretence. Eventually my mum could take no more and broke
the silence. Told everything. She explained what was going
on to my grandmother who had always been particularly con-
siderate and understanding. But she didn't get the sympathy
and support she was expecting. According to my grandmother,
my father's kind of behaviour was all you could ever expect
from a husband. My grandmother's husband had walked out
on her while she was giving birth to my father, and for as long
as anyone could remember, had led a secret life with another
woman, coming home at Christmas and pretending everything
was fine. She advised my mother to grin and bear it and not
be so neurotic. That this was a normal marriage. So much for
sisterly support. Of course the advice didn't work and my mother
continued to get worse. On Christmas day I drank a bottle of
vodka and passed out - unconsciousness seeming a far prefer-
able option to being awake. My grandmother died shortly after from a brain tumour, which probably helps to explain her
out-of-character response. At least I hope it does.

One day I returned from school to find out that my mother
was taking me back to England the next afternoon. No time
to think or question or argue. No time to say goodbye to friends,
except for one whose house I was packed off to for the night.
Someone did my packing for me. A silent drive down to Bos-
ton, my first time on a plane. The end of an episode. I remember

stepping onto the tarmac at Heathrow, six in the morning, that cold English chill reaching into my bones. Welcome home! We went to live in Bognor Regis. Home of Butlins and pasty-faced seaside day trippers, of old peoples homes and failed South London criminals. Sewage in the sea, arsehole of the South Coast.

I started at yet another new school, and having missed a year was unable to do the O-Levels I was interested in. Soon I was missing school more often than I attended. Life seemed to me as gloomy and dull as Bognor itself. Then I met a new set of friends, all much older than me, all into acid, speed and smoking dope. Many of them were friends of Leigh's (see LEIGH'S story in the book). It's funny we never met back then. We met fifteen years later on her first day working at Positively Women.

I remember my first fix. I was sitting in the living room of this big house where we'd all hang out. It was 1976, I remember because I was tripping on some Bicentennial acid (red, white and blue, like the American flag). As usual nothing much was happening and I was debating whether or not to go and look for some action elsewhere. Then this odd looking bloke turned up. He made a big entrance into the room so you couldn't miss the fact that he'd arrived, then started to empty out the contents of his pockets, looking for something, then looking for something else, making it clear he had important business to do. He proceeded to put some powder in a spoon, add water, heat it, draw it up into a syringe and shove it into his arm. I'd never seen anyone do it before, never seriously thought about doing it myself, but in my tripped out state of mind I thought it looked really 'beautiful'. I asked if he could do it for me but he didn't have any more powder. My friend Rick who was also tripping agreed it looked fun. He had some valium and we crushed them up and tried it out. Anyway that was the first time and even though the valium had no effect at least it was something new.

The next week the odd looking bloke (who later became a

best friend and then a dead-from-an-overdose best friend) turned up at my grandmother's where I was staying while she was away. He said he had a surprise for me. The surprise turned out to be a half ounce of amphetamine sulphate and a new syringe. He fixed me up with some after which I legged it to the toilet, threw up, then rushed back exclaiming joyfully that this was the best thing that had ever happened to me. We stayed there until we'd finished the whole half ounce. Pretty soon I did little else but buy, sell or shoot speed. Me and my mates, in my grandmother's house. Talking crap for days and days.

Jubilee year, 1977. Of the few memories I have of that summer, I remember Glastonbury festival, lying in a field off my face for a week. Selling speed to my dad's ex-students. Listening to the Sex Pistols in the park. And my first hit of morphine. I remember I hated that. My veins were bad by then and by the time I got the stuff in I'd lost half of it, blood all over my arms and feet and clotted in the spoon. I couldn't understand why everyone was raving about it, I was used to the rush and excitement of the speed, not the cosy, stoned silence of opiates. So I didn't bother too much with it, and in any case I was soon too ill with hepatitis and was back at my mother's convalescing. A few months later I moved out of home for good.

My brother and sister had returned to England shortly after my mother and I. From then on the nasty and drawn out divorce proceedings started. My dad wanted custody of them, but not me, which hurt a lot even though I didn't want to live with him. But it hurt none the less and reminded me that I was different and not really a part of the family. It proved in my mind that he hated me and partially blamed me for the marital breakup. In fact I was even used by my father as evidence that my mother was unfit to take care of her kids. When the case was heard in London mum won custody of all of us but my brother and sister had to go to the States on visits. I didn't.

Poor mum. She really did try her best but nothing she tried made any difference. I hardly saw Mathew and Rachel and when I did they were usually terrified. I made my eleven-year-old sister carry my drugs for me and hold the belt around my arm while I had a hit. At least it put her off ever trying it herself. My visits home were met with fear and anxiety, they never knew how I would disrupt their lives next. Generally there was a collective sigh of relief when I was no longer around.

Years later, when I finally felt ready to tell my mother that I was positive, I remember what she said. It took me back to that time and made me realize how things had changed and how I put such a different value on my life now, how I appreciated, loved, being alive. I no longer took it all for granted.

I told my mother that I was positive just before Christmas 1987, the year I was diagnosed. I hadn't felt ready to before and I was really scared when it actually came to doing it. The hardest bit about telling someone you love is dealing with their grief. Seeing the pain, fear and despair flash across their faces is the most terrible thing - you want to tell them not to worry but you know it will be there with them long after you've gone. My mother was in some ways more prepared than others, after all she was aware of all the drug stuff - we'd even spoken about the risks I'd taken, acknowledging the possibility. But suspecting is light years away from knowing and nothing can totally prepare you for that initial wave of confusion and disbelief. I arrived at lunch-time and tried to eat the meal she had prepared. Kept putting the fork down but no sound would come out of my mouth. Saying those words 'I'm positive' to someone you must tell is still as hard now as it was then, most of the time. Sometimes it gets easier.

Over coffee I say,
'Mum I've got something to tell you.'
She says,
'Oh no! You're not in trouble with the police are you?'
Me,
'No it's not that.'
Her,
'Oh well. Can't be that bad then.'

Me,

'I've had a blood test and I've got HIV.'

She pauses, looks thoughtful, then says to me,

'Well that doesn't mean you've got AIDS does it? You're perfectly healthy aren't you?'

I reply,

'Yes that's right mum. I'm fine.'

She tells me,

'Kate, when you were using every time you walked out through that door I'd say goodbye to you as if it were the last time. I never knew whether I'd ever see you alive again. Today you look the healthiest I've ever seen you. I know you'll be okay. If you ever need me I'll be here.'

Summer 1978 I met Richard. He was a con man and rip off artist but a real charmer who always got away with what no one else would have. By rights he should have been dead many times over, even then. He turned up last year when he saw my picture in an AIDS newsletter and made contact. I have to admire the man for making it this far. Maybe miracles really are possible. Anyway back then we spent a wild year together during which, from what I recall, our main and only aim was to consume whatever drug we could beg, borrow or steal, in as large a quantity as we could physically tolerate. Mainly heroin, morphine or dicanol. At some point during this period I woke up one morning and really understood what withdrawals were about.

Twelve months later we found ourselves on the boat to Amsterdam, Richard on the run from the law again. The money ran out after two days and the holiday was over. Back to making it pay on the streets. We got methadone prescriptions from five or six different doctors, sold most of it to buy heroin, ripped off tourists and bought too much cocaine. Sometimes we'd have a meal or a shower. Hard work but good money. The trouble is the more you make, the more you use, and you need more or the sicker you'll get. Always having to watch your back, be wary of your friends. It took me years of unlearning to trust people again. Once we sold a large amount of smack to some guys from Surinam. The only problem was that the 'friend' we'd scored it off had put some coins in the middle of the bag. Two and a half guilder pieces weigh a lot and when the guys found them they weren't too happy. They gave Richard two days to get the money back while they kept me in a room with a loaded gun by the exit. It never occurred to me until a long time after that there might have been any degree of danger involved. An underdeveloped sense of danger must be the premier qualification for a drug-using lifestyle.

Things got harder as the cold weather set in and the tourists were thinner on the ground; Richard and I fought all the time. I left Amsterdam and Richard in mid-winter. He followed me, got arrested and did time. I went back to chasing drugs across the South Coast and when he came out we just couldn't get along. I packed up and went to Morocco to put distance between us and clean up my act.

May 1991. Today my friend Anna died. I first met Anna back in 1979 when I was eighteen and living in Amsterdam. Richard and I used to buy drugs off her. Anna was concerned about me because I was throwing up all the time. I was getting thinner and weaker by the day. She suggested I might be pregnant and although I didn't believe it was possible, not having had a period for over two years, she persuaded me to get tested. As it turned out I was most definitely pregnant and Anna arranged for me to have an abortion.

I only saw Anna once or twice after that until ten years later when I was asked to visit a woman in hospital who had just been diagnosed with AIDS. It was Anna. This time I was in the position to offer support but the reversal of roles was odd. I had memories of her as this strong and together person who would take care of me. She was still strong in spirit, and remained so until her death, but her body was old and worn out. It scared me and brought back all those fears about my own health which I had struggled so hard to keep under control. The past was thrown right into the present in an unsettling way and unwanted, discarded memories involuntarily flooded back. For the next two years we kept in touch, saw each other sometimes, talked about old and new times and Anna hung on in there stubbornly refusing to let others tell her how to lead her life and refusing to die until she had sorted things out for her daughter. Now she's dead I feel angry at the loss of yet another life. At my personal loss of a link with my past which I had grown to be comfortable with. At the society which treated Anna and her daughter so badly towards the end. At the way that ten years into the pandemic the world is still not learning from it's mistakes. At the deaths to come.

Today I went to Anna's funeral. I need to be strong. But I don't feel strong. Others around me need to see me as being strong. It's hard but you become a good actor. Sometimes it's hard to stay optimistic when every month, every week, you see friends dying. I tell myself I must be optimistic, I must believe I will remain healthy. If not I will begin to think like a sick person, like a patient and thus become one. I feel under pressure to stay optimistic for others. Sometimes I feel like a fraud, a hypocrite. The words come out but there's no feeling behind them. How do we retain a positive approach without being in denial? Achieve a degree of acceptance without losing hope? I guess we must just keep working at it.

In 1980 - 81 I stayed in Morocco for nearly a year, working and then travelling for a while with friends. I loved it there and got well sorted out but was nevertheless ready to leave when I did. Back in England I reverted to my old habits for a while, then took off to Switzerland to run a bar for six months, clean up my act again and save some money. I was back in England for my twenty-first birthday. This time, to avoid getting into the same old scene again, I only stayed for a week before moving on.

My father and stepmother had recently moved out to San

Francisco and as we were getting on reasonably well by then, I went to visit, combining a chance to see them with the opportunity of exploring a city which I had heard and read so much about. From there I continued on down to Mexico for a few months. Meanwhile, I had a classic holiday romance - great drugs, great sex, and of course, back in those days, no clean needles or condoms. He left me with some happy memories, a cocktail of STDs, and another bout of hepatitis. I sometimes look back and wonder if it was then that I also contracted HIV. Not that it matters, but I suppose there's so much emphasis put on time in respect of disease progression and survival that so many of us get hung up on trying to work out exactly when we were infected.

Back to Amsterdam. This time I was making good money so I rented a beautiful flat and had all the drugs I needed or desired. I bumped into Richard again and he stayed at the flat for a while. One winter morning he pissed me off so much, I threw him out even though he wasn't all that well. Later that day he collapsed in the street and was rushed into hospital with pneumonia. Shortly after I was on a trip back home when I collapsed on my mother's kitchen floor screaming with pain and unable to move. It turned out I had pleurisy and pneumonia. I was grounded for some time and forced to stay at my mother's again while I recovered. The specialists at the local hospital were puzzled. I was not recovering properly and tests showed my immune system was shot to pieces. They told me that they believed I had some kind of virus but had no luck identifying it. Strangely, or maybe not so strangely, I have in later years come across several people I'd shared needles or had sex with around that time. We all had the same pneumonia. We are all HIV positive. Or dead. Why wouldn't they give us users clean needles when we were asking for them? How many lives might have been saved?

Recovered from the pneumonia, I still had some money saved so I decided perhaps now was the time to fulfil an old fantasy of going to India. Romantically, I hoped that being there would teach me something of myself, of my father's culture, of a part of me that had been cut off since birth. In fact what it taught me was that I could never be more than an outsider in that culture. That my culture was middle-class European. End of story. Less romantically, I knew I could get cheap drugs there.

I purchased a guide book and an airline ticket, found a friend to come with me and we set off. I remember fixing my last quarter gram in the toilets at Heathrow Airport before checking in and then being pulled apart at the baggage check, completely off my face. By the time we reached Bombay we'd linked up with some hard-core travellers who knew all the ropes. Within two hours of our arrival we'd scored a couple of grams of smack outside the hotel and were slumped in the bedroom, comfortably stoned and oblivious to the noise and colour of the strange and different world outside. Within two months I was using a couple of grams of smack a day and remained continuously stoned until I finally departed nearly two years later.

My adventures from this trip could fill a book of their own but to cut a long story short, I arrived back in England facing charges of possession and importation of heroin. I had two choices - either to stay and face the music and get locked up for a long time, or to run away again. It was as if I'd been running away for years. From facing myself or others, from making any real decisions or changes, from taking a good look at any reality that did not incorporate taking heroin. Once my back was against the wall, I knew I really did want to stop. I knew I could break the circle and stay clean for good. I knew I had to and was ready to do it. I just wasn't sure how. What I did know was how I didn't want to stop. No rehabs or prison medical wings for me; I knew that if anyone forced me to stop it wouldn't last. I had to do it for myself and it had to be my choice and my achievement alone.

So I left England yet again for Paris, where a journalist friend of mine was living. By now I had cut down to using only a quarter gram a day and during the first week there I cut down even more. Then I stopped. And I never started again. At the time, when I was going through all the discomfort and withdrawal, I didn't realize the full extent to which my life was about to change. That this was such a turning point, only to became apparent to me much later on.

When I was over the worst, I travelled to the South of France to stay with some friends I'd met in India. They knew about my situation and offered to let me stay for as long as I needed. They worked on the markets in the area and always needed help with their stalls. I ended up working with them for several months. I needed to be with people who were not users and to be filling my days from morning till night with physical work that tired me out each day, leaving me no time to think about trying to score. I became fit, brown and healthy and succeeded in staying clean. By winter time the Cote d'Azur was relatively quiet, empty and cold. The markets were no longer crowded by tourists and the money not so good.

I decided to try my luck back in Paris. A friend of my friend had a small self-contained room above her flat which she let me have for next to no rent and I set out to find work. Again I fell on my feet when I was introduced to a group of rich Parisian lesbians who all wanted someone to run errands for them. I got enough work this way to survive and to go out in the evenings, and to put some money aside. My first and favourite was Monique, who was a mad, alcoholic, speed freak psychoanalyst. I went round every morning, Monday through Friday, stopping to buy croissants on the way. Three of them. One for her, one for me, and one for her mad dog who would sink its teeth into whatever it spotted coming through the door first, so I had to make sure it was the croissant and not me! My task was to dispose of all the whisky bottles, beer cans and cigarette butts, jam the pile of clothes into a cupboard and transform the place into a consulting room before they returned. Once they were back and the patients began to arrive, I tackled the chaos elsewhere.

That winter was bitterly cold and my room had no heating. When she could, my sister saved up her dole money and came over. One evening, lying in my single bed, huddled together fully clothed to keep warm and having polished off a bottle of cooking brandy, we decided to go to California to find some sunshine.

We both went out and stayed at my dad and stepmother's for six months and worked at the usual, illegal, shitty jobs. It wasn't till I arrived there that it really hit me what a mess I was in emotionally. After years of trying to block out thoughts and emotions it was the first time I'd allowed myself any space to think. It was the nearest I've come to a total breakdown but I guess that's not too surprising considering all the lost time I had to make up for.

Thinking back it's hard to describe what I was going through. All I knew was drugs. Since the age of fifteen there had been little else. Nothing I had done, no place I had been had any meaning outside of the context of my using. My whole identity was built around being a user, the way I perceived myself, the way others perceived me. All the status, the respect and the power I had was non-existent outside of that narrow world. I put down the 'straight world', thus reinforcing the validity of what I was doing and justifying it to myself at the same time. And from a different perspective this was what the straight world did to me as a drug user.

It wasn't the physical aspect of giving up drugs that was hardest, but rather having to learn the rules and codes of conduct in a world where the central focus and point of contact was not drugs. When the old world had gone, I no longer knew who I was, I had no clear purpose in life. Like Sleeping Beauty waking up after many years and finding that the world has moved on but she's been left behind. Her only recollections of the intervening years are dreams which she cannot communicate to the inhabitants of this world. Their logic or form hold no relevance. She soon learns not to refer to these dreams. They make people uncomfortable and suspicious. She realizes that to fit in she must reinvent herself as someone new, find a history which others can relate to and accept. This Sleeping Beauty almost didn't make it.

I returned to Europe, to Paris, Amsterdam, and then back to Paris again. During my six months in the USA, I'd laid a good many old ghosts to rest, done a lot of accepting and rejecting, and growing up. Haunted by old nightmares in which I was always being chased, running away from something I feared, it became clear to me that there was one major hurdle left before the slate was wiped. It meant going back to England and dealing with my outstanding charges.

I had a solemn dinner with friends near where the bus left. It felt like the Last Supper. They saw me on to the coach promising to call my mother's the next day to see if I'd made it through immigration at Dover without being arrested. The night boat was near empty and I sat alone in the bar save for two truck drivers. I never needed a quarter bottle of brandy like the one I drank that night with those drivers. Six in the morning at Dover, I walked through, no questions asked.

The prospect of spending Christmas and New Year locked up didn't hold much appeal, so to avoid that possibility I hid out at my mum's till the festivities were over. In the New Year I contacted my solicitor and he arranged for me to go in and be charged. Fortunately he also managed to get me out on bail after only one night in the cells. I knew I had to pull out all the stops if things were to go my way in court, so I set to work fast. I moved to London and found a 'socially responsible' job working with people with learning difficulties. I started an Access course which guaranteed me a place at university on completion; I submitted to endless social enquiry reports and medical reports and blood tests and regular signing on at the police station. At this time I met and became friends with some of the most brilliant people I've ever known. They remain my closest friends today and have been there for me through everything. These, and my friendships in France, were the only ones since my early teens that weren't solely based on drugs. With them I learned to appreciate things which had never seemed important before. I learned the value of real friendship.

When my case was finally heard, my hard work paid off. I was looking at a 90 per cent chance of at least two years, and had everything prepared for that eventuality. As it turned out, I received a two years suspended sentence, a mega fine and two years' probation. In the same way that you never appreciate life as keenly as when you're confronted with death, you never appreciate your freedom so much as when you stand to lose it. We went out to celebrate and I was still celebrating the next year when I went for an HIV test.

When my results came back negative I was told off by the doctor. I was 'an hysterical woman, wasting NHS resources. Women don't get AIDS.' Oh no?

A week later I was summoned back to the clinic. They'd made some sort of mistake over the results, the letter that popped through my letter-box on a Friday night explained. 'Mistake? What mistake?' I asked myself and my friends during the long days until the clinic was next open. Giving me someone else's results was the mistake they'd made. 'Well, these things will happen. No one's to blame. You have antibodies to the human immunodefficiency virus. Do you understand what this means?'

Walking out of the clinic after my results, this is what I remember. Everything else is lost. I remember leaving the hospital, clutching a handful of leaflets. I remember turning the corner of Holloway Road onto Seven Sisters to catch a 253 bus to Finsbury Park. I remember seeing faces but they seem far away, or rather I do. A million miles away from anyone else on the planet. Looking down on a cardboard cut-out of me, walking. In the real world, but not a part of it. Next I'm walking down the road where Peter G's house is but I've gone too far. I must have changed onto a 106 bus, got off and walked too far. I walk back, into the garden, and knock on the kitchen door. I'm in the kitchen and I start laughing hysterically. 'You know that test I had? Well it was positive.' Peter G goes to take a bath. When he comes back, he's been crying. Then I'm in a health shop on Upper Street. Peter N is with me. I buy live yoghurt and drink it from the carton because it's good for me. We are in Sisterwrite bookshop, looking for books on AIDS, can't remember if we find any. Then in Gays The Word for the same reason. I need to find an answer. Some time later, the first time on my own, I sit in my room, on the end of my bed, looking in the mirror. I see a dying person and I cry and cry some more. Somehow familiar. Two weeks of my life. This is what I remember. Every thing else is lost.

PETER G'S MEMORIES

When someone remembers an extremely challenging experience, accurately, it is easier to colour the memory with adjustment and appropriate understanding. When I learnt that Kate was HIV positive, I was terrified and it was not an elusive fear. I was terrified for her, me, my friends and the world, in no particular order. I was numb even though the acute inadequacy of Kate's doctor had left us all for three days without certainty. In fact, I had felt even vaguer than that suggests. It would not happen to her.

That day, that Wednesday, I began to live with the horrible fact that information about this virus was negligible. And that was deliberate. My intense ignorance at that time is embarrassing and painful to remember. I did know what it was and I knew my distance from it, and as a gay man I knew about the lies. I knew nothing else. I did not know that Kate's body had been living with the virus for who knows how long. I had no idea about the progress from HIV to AIDS. AIDS was what she had. She was not HIV positive, she had AIDS and she would die - that's what I believed at the time.

I went to work that day and someone described how a friend had been shot at a party. I then told her about Kate. I felt ashamed because I know I was thinking about myself as much as, if not more, than my friend, never mind the friend of my colleague. As the afternoon progressed I kept thinking, we need to know more. I was all emotion, but rational enough to focus on the fact that somehow, this was Kate's personal conclusion of a lifestyle that involved sharing needles for however long it was.

*Simply, I knew that I would not do as much as I should for my
friend, and that deep down I was as selfish as I had hoped I was
not. So, I pitied Kate, and I pitied myself that day, that week,
which was not very constructive.*

I'd had a fling with Jools the year before I found out. I felt that
I'd been used in an attempt to revive a failing relationship which
he'd been involved in for the previous four years - make the
other partner jealous and they'll come back to you. I enjoyed
the affair for what it was: no demands, expectations or strings
attached. It kind of fizzled out but not in an unpleasant way.
We stayed friends, socialized, worked and even went on holiday
together.

By the time I was diagnosed we were no longer working in
the same place and were in contact far less frequently than before - so it was quite unusual for me to phone him. I left it about
a week before I felt in any way ready to break the news to him,
and when I finally did call he told me he was off on holiday
the next day. Of course there was no way I could tell him before he went (imagine what a holiday that would have been!),
so I said I'd ring when he got back. He sounded suspicious
and rather concerned that something was wrong but I reasoned
that a little suspense and intrigue to dwell on while on holiday
was far better than the reality of my news.

When he came home I called and we arranged for him to
come over. I was scared shitless that morning and bought a
half bottle of brandy. I had a few excessive anticipatory slurps
before he arrived and as soon as he walked through the door I
poured two enormous glasses of the stuff. I reckon he guessed
at that moment. I told him pretty matter-of-factly (how else does
one do it?) - not knowing how he'd respond. Jools is a nice
guy so I didn't exactly expect him to start screaming at me or
anything like that. He just asked if I was all right, never mind
about him, how was I doing?

As always it was impossible to divine what he was really
feeling at that moment - Jools has never been one to show

emotion. He told me that he'd guessed what I had to say anyway - which made me feel even worse. I'll always appreciate
his outwardly caring and generous response - it's difficult to
put into words how much it meant to me at that time and how
much it made me feel better about myself and about the world.

I arranged for him to go to the clinic. My feelings were
confusingly mixed. On the one hand I dreaded having given
it to him; I feared his resentment, feared that he would hate
me, that his relationship with Monica would suffer, even that
she might be infected. I didn't know how I could live with that
guilt. On the other hand, part of me, a guilty and ashamed part
of me, hoped that Jools would be positive too. Now, looking
back, I no longer feel so bad about having wished this. I'm glad
that Jools was not infected but I understand why I felt what I
did. I saw my future as bleak and lonely. I believed that if Jools
tested positive, then perhaps we could get back together and
support each other.

Jools got his results and he was negative. He came straight
from the hospital to tell me, but he didn't stay long. I think we
both felt awkward and didn't really know what to say to each
other. He left to go and celebrate and I was left feeling like
the brave and tragic heroine in a film.

JOOLS' MEMORIES
*May 1987. We'd just booked our flight to Rome, or rather I
had - that was the way our relationship was going. I did all
the organizing and left the emotions to Monica. I provided the
stable, ever present partner. This was the way it had been for
three years: we were a mature couple, we said we could handle
each others' affairs, but really I couldn't, I hated it. Oh well,
that's what being a modern couple is all about. Around this time
Monica had 'renounced her immature past and was willing to
commit herself to me'. Great ! Finally I was enough, I was her
partner and she was in love with me, forsaking all others. It
was all the more unusual then, that on the eve of our depar-
ture Kate should ring me.*

Kate and I had had an affair, it was good. It all ended so well from my point of view. Best of all, we were friends, shared acquaintances and she was an escape from my incestuous social scene.

What, I thought, was so important that she couldn't discuss it over the phone? Arrogantly, I thought it was my advice she wanted, something shady or illegal maybe.

Rome was a last gasp holiday: the thrill of our relationship had gone - it went as soon as there was no competition. I didn't want her any more; we didn't have sex. Every step around Rome I knew I was HIV positive and was dying - such was the level of my ignorance about HIV infection. I wanted to get home and see Kate to confirm my fears. I felt such a martyr - I could handle and say nothing, even to Monica. Already it was I, me, myself, mine, me.

So I met Kate and, yes, I was sent to the clinic. I had no thought for Kate's feelings, no thanks for the courage it had taken to tell me face to face, after all I'd suffered for a week already hadn't I?

Peter, my wonderful counsellor, was very concerned, or at least his main concern was whether I'd tell my parents or not - this was before I'd even had the test!

Gloves on, needle in, blood out and three weeks wait if you please. I'm so glad I pay for the NHS. 'For God's sake! I want to know now!'

This little account has been very impersonal, cynical, fatalistic, until now. Those three weeks are the most inhuman punishment known to cosseted Britons. Privately I'd know tomorrow, but on the NHS I have to wait three weeks to know my sentence. I defy anyone to think anything but selfishly during that period. I had no thoughts for Kate who already knew. I wondered how to reconcile my nonexistent feelings for Monica with the predicament into which I, maybe, had led her. I read all there was about HIV and ARC, deriving hope from the positive articles and despair from Sun-style paranoid reports. Above all I knew I was in limbo, in ignorance - I thought, in three weeks I will know whether I will die sooner or later.

You've probably noticed by now very little reference to my feelings toward the woman who could have inadvertently given me the virus; I'm very sorry to say that I had very few. Selfishness ruled my thoughts. There was no bitterness, no anger, no judgement, but worst, no empathy. Assuming I was positive, I planned ahead, how to enjoy the rest of my life - I even thought that, at last, the council would give me a flat - a bell that rang true for me, but rings hollow for those who need it so much more.

Three weeks passed. It was three weeks that did not change my life. At her request I went to see Kate first. She gave me a half bottle of brandy, Chivas Regal - I'll never forget it. Then I waited sweating in the rotting prefab. I envied the others who probably only had some nasty dose or another. Then came my summons.

'Next please, Mr Hesketh.' Oh God!

I walked in, didn't recognize the doctor - nice to have a familiar face. You could hear everything in the waiting room. The unknown doctor looked at my notes and then triumphantly held up my negative result.

'Well done, Mr Hesketh. You've passed, and with flying colours! See you next time. Next please.'

With a slap on the back I was off down the Holloway Road at 80 mph - well, I'd nearly died anyway. Then came the moment no words can ever describe - I took the Chivas Regal and my liberated, joyful soul to the woman who had selflessly and courageously told me. We embraced, but it was a cold embrace for there could never be a wider gap in emotions - only writing this now can I imagine the sickness in her heart at that moment. We exchanged pleasantries and I left to lead the rest of my life.

I swore to myself to support Kate in any way she wanted and to use my experience to challenge complacent and judgemental heterosexual attitudes. As ever, I did, and I do, nothing.

In a strange way my life has only felt special during those three weeks when I thought I was positive, when death was no longer a fear, life became a reality.

OCTOBER 1990

When I asked Jools to write about how he felt when I was diagnosed it was two and a half years after the event. For some
reason I was always angry with him and whatever he said or
did, I would invariably find fault with it - a word or a glance
would be sufficient for me to feel critical and superior. I would
always be sarcastic or cynical, there was always some excuse.
Because we'd never talked about how either of us felt, or what
effect my diagnosis had had on us and on our friendship, I never
really knew where I stood, and this made me nervous and defensive when we were together. I wondered how he felt about
me now; I dreaded his sympathy. I was afraid he might regret
we'd ever been together.

With my other close friends, I'd talked through all this - we'd
been through the whole thing together and come out the other
side, our friendship strengthened by the journey. Jools and I
were no longer close to each other, and yet, when I had first
heard my results he had been the first person I thought of.

Strangely enough Jools and Peter G became best mates, and
it was really through Peter G that Jools and I became reac-
quainted. As always, I met up with Peter regularly, and from
time to time he'd update me on Jools. So I knew that Jools and
Peter planned a trip to Africa and one of us suggested we all
get together, along with my sister Rachel, prior to their depar-
ture.

I don't know what happened that night or why but while Peter
and Rachel chatted, Jools and I talked. We talked like we'd
never done: we said what we needed to say. So much unfinished
business - concluded at last.

I see him a lot now. We'll meet up for lunch or at a friends
or he'll come round to my place. Sometimes I just call him up
for a chat or gossip. He's a friend - I feel closer to him than I
ever did before. I hope he feels the same.

After my diagnosis I remember being obsessed by this passage out of a book by Don Dellilo:

'Death has entered. It is inside you. You are said to be dying and yet are separate from the dying, can ponder it at your leisure, literally see it on the x-ray photograph or computer screen the horrible alien logic of it all. It is when death is rendered graphically, is televised so to speak, that you sense an eerie separation between your condition and yourself. A network of symbols has been introduced, an awesome technology wrested from the gods. It makes you feel like a stranger in your own dying.'

I felt, as he says elsewhere, like:

'I've got death inside me - it's just a question of whether I can outlive it or not.'

It was as if I had a time bomb inside me. The virus/the bomb retained it's own identity, apart from me, yet a part of me too. It was not merely a simple strip of DNA but the real and physical manifestation of an ongoing moral/ideological/physical/medical/political battle. My body had become the battlefield.

I decided to fight the virus any way I could. The trouble was I didn't know how. It seemed that no book could tell me. It made sense to try and keep fit so I became ultra-obsessed with my physical health. I visited a naturopath who put me on a strict diet and recommended vitamin supplements. I gave up smoking and started working out each morning. I gave up drinking and stopped going out. Increasingly my social life became impossible. I couldn't go out to dinner because of my diet. If I went to the pub or out clubbing I became resentful and irritated with my friends for getting drunk. I felt excluded. I was always reminded why I was denying myself everything I liked, and I felt a distance emerging between myself and my friends because they were not going through what I was. I was utterly miserable. Eventually I realized that this way was not for me. So I stopped being so rigid about things, had the odd drink, got drunk sometimes, continued to eat reasonably well but indulged in junk food when I wanted, started smoking again. Once I managed to find that balance I felt better and had a whole lot more fun. Sometimes the balance tips one way, sometimes the other, but I've learnt to listen to the signals my body is sending me and adjust my actions accordingly. To be more in tune. I realized that the quality of life and being happy is more important than living for a long time and being miserable.

Another way I fought the virus was by arming myself with information. The more informed, the more I felt I could control my situation. The trouble was that when I did find material to read it was all so conflicting that it made it hard to know what to believe. That was the hardest - realizing that no one knew all the answers, perhaps no one knew any of them. For me, learning to live with and accept so many uncertainties was, and continues to be, the major challenge.

I also fought the virus by TALKING ABOUT IT. I was fortunate in that I could talk to my friends. I never even considered trying to hide my results from them. I believed, and still do, that if I cannot be upfront with someone about such a major issue in my life then we cannot have a genuinely open and honest relationship. The gay men I knew were well aware that they could quite easily have been diagnosed. Being positive was a possibility we'd all talked about a lot in the past and I just happened to be the one who decided to take the test. So talking about it was not anything new, but the knowledge that we had gained made everything more real and immediate to us. The more I was able to talk about it, the less mystery and fear surrounded it for me.

Yet another way I fought the virus was through my involvement with Positively Women. Being in contact with other women living with the virus gave me access to a special and unique kind of support. It helped me gain a measure of hope and optimism for the future and an acceptance which did not incorporate fatalism or passivity. As time went on I recognized how my involvement helped to sustain and keep me going; I was taking an active role in my relationship to the virus while at the same time not letting it dominate my life.

KATE

PETER N'S MEMORIES

It's fast approaching five years since I first came across a woman who had been diagnosed as HIV positive. In fact it was probably the first time that I had actually been in close contact with anyone who knew that they were positive. I had heard of many people who had died from AIDS. But I never knew that they were positive. In those days you never knew until someone had died or was on their deathbed.

Kate was the closest friend of my then boyfriend. I didn't know her that well. I lived in Manchester and came to London to visit my lover on alternate weekends.

It is strange how one's ignorance becomes most apparent the nearer one is to a subject. I thought that I was fairly well clued up on AIDS. After all I was busy around the gay scene, knew that AIDS was fast becoming a major tragedy and had read bits and pieces here and there. So I thought that I was as informed as most people. In fact I knew next to nothing. Which was about as informed as most other people were.

Kate walked into my boyfriend's flat one Thursday midmorning. Peter and I were having a cup of tea. I had arrived from Manchester the previous evening and we had spent the night in drunken delight at each other's company. Kate didn't bounce in in her usual style and Peter seemed to know why. I was bemused, there was obviously something that they both knew that I didn't. Kate walked towards Peter and from his seated position he put his arms around her hips. She burst into tears and said that the result was positive. I still didn't know what was going on. I didn't know about Kate's drug using past, or if I did I hadn't given it much thought.

As I watched Kate in Peter's arms and could sense the tears falling down her cheeks, things suddenly began to dawn on me. Oh my God! My stomach began to churn with fear. All of a sudden I didn't understand anything about AIDS. What did it mean that this woman stood before me had this virus rushing around her body? It didn't mean anything. HIV was an abstract concept, something you read about in the gay press. One read it like a horror story, a fiction that frightens but doesn't touch. AIDS was what killed people who had just disappeared from the gay scene one day. You would contemplate what it meant and it wouldn't really mean anything. Not then.

Directly in front of me was this women who had just told my lover that she was HIV positive. I was there, it was real and I didn't know what to do. Or that I should or could do anything. What I did know, however, was that she needed her friends now more than ever. I didn't know how or why or what. I just knew that I had to help her with this thing in any way she wanted.

She had an awful experience at the hospital. They had told her that they couldn't do anything for her. They just said 'Don't get pregnant. The baby could be born infected'. They talked to her in medical jargon about the virus, advised her to take up weight training, and to stop smoking. That was it, she was expected to walk out of there and get on with the rest of her life. She was sent to see a male counsellor who didn't seem to know what he was doing, as many didn't then, and nobody told her what she wanted to know. All she wanted to know was how to maintain her health.

We had always had a mistrust of the medical profession and since nobody, doctor or otherwise, was very sure about this new disease, we trusted them even less. As a result, we were interested in alternative ways of preventing ill health for someone who is HIV positive. This was our first course of action. Kate and I went off the next day in search of information about ways of keeping healthy in the light of being HIV positive. We had no idea where to begin, but we decided that bookshops were as good a place as any. Down into town we went. The most obvious starting point was Gays the Word bookshop. We found such delightful advice as: eat, eat, eat as many Mars bars as you can possibly get down your neck. Energy is what you need, so the easiest form was sugar and carbohydrates. Not quite what we expected. Not quite the holistic approach to health that we *favoured. Off we went again. This time to Dillons bookshop. There, after searching all over the building for the 'AIDS section', we found a much larger collection of books. None the less the health information was the same. We began to despair and I realized my ignorance of the AIDS issue, again. But more importantly we realized how little information there was about a holistic approach to being HIV positive. Kate decided that the best thing to do was to look for general information about preventative health care. She gathered knowledge of vitamin supplements and minerals as well as the particular qualities of certain foodstuffs like garlic - as an antibiotic.*

We needed to find other women who were HIV positive because Kate wanted to deal with some of the isolation and alienation that she was feeling. This proved extremely difficult at first. At one point I telephoned the Terrence Higgins Trust and was told that the only woman contact was on holiday and that if I gave details they would get her to ring back. No one ever contacted her. This made me, let alone Kate, begin to feel that she would be just left in a swirl of uncertainty, not knowing when this dreadful thing would suddenly explode from the seemingly quiet recesses of her body, when she would one day wake up looking just like the photographs that we had seen in the press of thin, gaunt and wasting bodies.

I remember the first time that I actually got a glimpse of how this situation made Kate feel. She told me that one day she had woken up and could see herself in the mirror at the end of her bed. She described how she looked at herself and then suddenly burst into tears and began to pull at her hair in thorough hatred of herself and despair at the seeming inevitability of death. This shocked and frightened me. I felt that this was not right, that no matter what, another human being shouldn't be made to feel like this. But the only information we had at that time said categorically that at some point, if you were antibody positive you would die a horrible death. Without question. At this point people weren't dealing with larger issues about mortality and other belief systems.

One day Kate was looking through a listings magazine and came across a group of women who were HIV positive and looking for other women like themselves. She contacted them and that was the beginning of Positively Women.

Kate threw herself into the world of HIV and AIDS. For the first time the politics of AIDS began to dawn on me. Through Kate I realized that there were intense political issues resulting from the lack of attention to this epidemic. The paltry information and misinformation had huge consequences for the ways in which people were led to view their lives and bodies. Through our friendship, I have learnt that there seems to be a plot to establish that HIV equals death. I have learnt that there is simply no such inevitability. I have been able to merge the politics involved with HIV and AIDS with my own world view. Learned to deal with the prospect of my own HIV status, what it means to not know. From day one, gay men have been tormented by the possibility that they might be positive. Every cold, every ache, every blemish was interpreted as an indication that they were positive. My friendship with Kate has helped me realize that positive or not, we have to take responsibility for our own bodies.

Kate set about helping other women to come to terms with a positive diagnosis or letting them know that they were not the only one. She and her colleagues constantly reiterate the specific needs that women who are HIV positive face. Constantly reiterate the need for the World Health Organisation, the governments of powerful nations, the huge multinational pharmaceutical conglomerates, and the boy next door to understand that this is a universal health crisis that is not confined to particular groups who are hell bent on poisoning the great white male. God forbid.

By the time I finally made contact with Positively Women (back then just Sheila and one other woman) I had finished my Access course and was waiting to begin at university in the autumn. I was determined that my positive result was not going to stop me from carrying on 'life as normal,' or changing my existing plans. I began to study for my degree, but at the same time got caught up in my activities around the group, until two years on, at the end of my second year, I decided that my priority was to work full-time for Positively Women. During those two years of growing involvement I also went through the gradual and difficult process of telling the members of my family about my status and about what I was doing.

My sister Rachel was the first family member I told. She is the closest one to me. There's no way I could keep a secret from her. I told her the first time I saw her after I'd found out. She came to visit for the weekend with her new boyfriend, Sean, and as she walked through the door she asked me what it was. I laughed and felt embarrassed for Sean. I told her and laughed some more but there were tears in my eyes which I was fighting back. The awkwardness and absurdity of saying it in front of a total stranger made the whole situation all the more bizarre and unreal, but in a funny kind of way it also made it easier.

RACHEL'S MEMORIES

Any retrospective account is open to reconstruction, not least an account of a traumatic event. It feels strange to be asked to recount my reactions when told my sister was ·HIV positive, as it was a story I had never told as something with a beginning and an end. Yet it is a story that is often present in my mind, below the surface and not made explicit, a collection of unstructured feelings. When trying to write this I was conscious that I was imposing order on experiences that I had not openly resolved. My strongest memory is of a physical feeling, the type of internal convulsion you get when your body takes the brunt of what your mind cannot accept. Kate was nervous and giggly - I knew that she had a secret, or something important that she wasn't telling me. I naturally drew her into our sisterly banter in order to extract the gossip. I knew that it wasn't something trivial, I immediately thought that she must be pregnant. I kept pushing, what was it? She told me.

Defence mechanisms locked in the mind, I felt an overwhelming need not to cry. Kate had tears in her eyes but wasn't crying; in fact I seem to remember that she was still softly giggling. I decided at that point that if she didn't cry, nor would I. My boyfriend was in the room at the time and I was glad because I couldn't imagine telling him what I had just heard. I couldn't look at him, I avoided his eyes which I knew would show shock and upset. I could only look at Kate. I wanted to shut out the rest of the world. I didn't want anyone to ask me if I was all right, I couldn't afford to ask myself that question. I hadn't had the time to think about what it meant, to try and understand and therefore to know how to put myself back together again.

When I was younger I often imagined myself at the funerals of loved ones, picturing myself in the centre stage receiving flowers and attention. Another reoccurring daydream had me looking beautiful in a hospital bed, terminally ill with tuberculosis. There would always be a trail of selected visitors, tearfully admitting their true feelings for me and their despair when faced with losing me. Of course I always miraculously recovered. I suddenly felt very guilty about these fantasies. I had to make sure I didn't demand attention and sympathy from others, it no longer seemed romantic that someone was dying. I didn't want to tell anyone about Kate, I was scared about my ulterior motives. For once I didn't want a drama. My guilt about these daydreams passed, they no longer feel like dark secrets. I suppose they are easily understood, ways of dealing with mortality and insignificance. I have found that trying to 'understand' both one's own reactions and the virus itself, whilst not resolving the situation, enables you to regain some of the control that was swept away by nature and fate when you hear that someone you love is HIV positive and could die of AIDS.

I carried on that weekend in a myopic state putting all my energy into trying to act normal and avoiding real contact with everyone except Kate. I kept on looking at her, overly conscious that she might not always be there.

The next stage, which must be a classic response to such a crisis, was a desperate need to find out more about the disease. I couldn't ask Kate 'are you going to die?' I couldn't even form that question in my own head. Kate gave me a book which I read, then another and another and another. The more I read the more I could deal with the knowledge, as it was abstracted from the direct personal pain.

I was never shocked that Kate was HIV positive. I had realized before that it was a possibility, but I was disappointed and angry that it was a reality. Suddenly an invisible virus had come into a delicately reformed life with a crushing impersonal effect.

There are many ways that this initial knowledge has become part of everyday life for me. There are occasions which are symbolic landmarks: sharing cake with the same fork, finally crying myself into exhaustion, writing this. Yet there is also a continuity of feeling - I still take strength from watching Kate as she lives a normal life with the virus within her and the way that she is able to motivate herself and others.

If Kate dies I will probably fall to pieces and feel the pain of mourning in full, no matter how long I have had to prepare for it. That will happen when it happens, if it happens. Until then both Kate and I are living everyday lives. I don't feel as though I am waiting any more, but nor am I hiding from it.

'We can wait another hour if you like. We can become friends then. Or we can wait until closing time. We can become friends then. Or we can wait until tomorrow, only that means that you must come in here tomorrow and perhaps you have something else to do.... Tell me - what is this thing about time? Why is it better to be late than early? People are always saying, we must wait, we must wait. What are they waiting for?' James Baldwin.

There is an underlying sense of urgency which has permeated all aspects of my life. Waiting is a luxury which perhaps I can no longer afford and which I certainly no longer desire. In my personal vocabulary waiting used to mean patience - now it means complacency or chances not taken.

Many claim (or hope) that AIDS has put the romance back into sex: courtship, 'commitment', 'getting to know each other', or even marriage (if you're heterosexual) before you fuck. For me it has meant the opposite. My sex life has become for the most part, distinct from my emotional life. Sex fulfils a physical need, only emotional in that I have a need for physical contact, while my social life and friendships are more intense, more honest and more valued since my diagnosis and fulfil my emotional needs. The two rarely overlap.

I used to be a great romantic, only sleeping with people I 'really cared about'. Now I'd usually rather have a one night stand. A stranger I'll probably not see again. No complications. No traumatic time consuming and energy draining relationships. No stress. No hurt or rejection. Just sex for the pure enjoyment of it. I like it better this way.

Maybe the necessity of discussing safer sex with my partners has resulted in more experimentation and discovery of what I like, but it's also about becoming more confident and assertive as time goes on.

But for a long time after I was diagnosed I felt completely asexual. The implicit, and sometimes explicit, messages about people with HIV which I saw on the television, in newspapers and magazines, in AIDS leaflets, and on the lips of many health care professionals and *Sun* readers alike, told us that we were diseased, infectious, a threat to the 'general population', and as such had a duty not to have sex or reproduce. As for enjoying sex, well we had no right to enjoy something that was so wrong. The only emotion we were rightfully entitled to was one of guilt. The result being that an old self destructive streak reared it's ugly head again, this time in the form of compulsive eating. A consequence of this constant binging was that I put on weight, felt full of self-hatred, unattractive and, therefore, sexually unavailable. This enabled me to protect myself against having to confront a lot of tricky emotional issues. Then there was the fear of having to tell someone my status. The fear of saying those words out loud. The fear of rejection. However, not having sex also meant letting those messages and voices win. It was not celibacy chosen for the right reasons, but rather enforced by the psychological bullying and propaganda of ignorant individuals and governments. An odd and distressing predicament to be in. On the one hand, wanting to have sex if only to affirm my right to do so, to proclaim my belief in the falsity of those messages, on the other hand, anger at myself for having, however unwillingly, absorbed and internalized those messages to such a degree that I couldn't bring myself to sleep with anyone.

Eventually I did sleep with someone who already knew. Shock that it didn't matter to them, that they weren't afraid of contamination, that they didn't look at me and only see a disease. Once was all it took and the spell was broken, like being a virgin. Ever since it's kept getting better!

Everyone is talking about safer sex, yet it's amazing how seldom they practise it. The problem seems to be that the only language we have with which to talk about sex immediately objectifies and distances us from our own experience. Too often we put off talking and rely on an underdeveloped sense of each other's body language. As far as I am aware I am not particularly skilled in the art of mind-reading and neither are my partners. So we're constantly making assumptions about what the other likes based solely upon a few 'oohs' or 'aahs' or on previous experience. We all know it's stupid, that we should be talking, that we probably could be enjoying sex more if we did so. Yet we're afraid or embarrassed to break the silence.

For me, as a woman who sleeps with men, there is the condom problem. Although I don't see it as a necessarily essential component of good sex, I do enjoy fucking, so therefore I need and want my partners to use condoms for several obvious reasons: I don't want to get pregnant; I don't want to become re-infected with HIV; I don't want to get any other STDs; I don't want to infect, or re-infect my partner; when we use a condom it feels like we're being good to ourselves and to each other. I feel safer and happier when we use a condom. So how come there's a problem?

Here from (very occasional) past experience are some excuses for not using or not wanting to use a condom: some men don't want to use them, even though they always know I'm positive; you're both too drunk or stoned to care; you get too 'carried away' and don't want to lose that 'spontaneity' (usually when you're too drunk or stoned to care about the potential consequences); it feels 'better' without one (which is debatable when weighed up against the good reasons to use a condom; still, it's usually the man's line anyway); neither of you will take responsibility for stopping, getting one out and putting it on (again back to the problem of communication or rather the lack of it): danger and risk taking can be exciting, so can doing things you're not supposed to be doing; you've run out (at least this means you HAVE been using them).

The first list is about the rational sensible me, the one usually in control and making the decisions. The second list represents the 'oh just this once' part of me. It's about a different rationale, which for whatever reasons, operates outside the context of AIDS prevention strategies. It's hard to admit that you have had unsafe sex, especially if you're positive. There's a lot of moralizing going on about the responsibility of HIV positive individuals to protect the health of those who are not infected, and far too little talk of responsibility on all sides, for us ALL, no matter what our status, to protect and care for each other and for ourselves. Most of us don't always practise what we preach all of the time but if we aren't able to be honest about and talk about why, then nothing will change. In many circumstances there may be as equally rational reasons for having unsafe as safer sex - especially for many women (the desire to get pregnant, lack of power or control over the situation, and so on). We must begin to examine and understand these contexts both on a personal level as sexually active individuals in the 1990s and on a larger scale if health education and AIDS prevention are to succeed.

LUCY'S LETTER

October 24, 1991

Dear Kate,

I'm sorry that I couldn't respond to your question right away about how I felt when you came to San Francisco and told your father and me about you being HIV positive. But here I am now, a few weeks later, wanting to give you my version. I warn you, I am no more perfect in this recollection than I usually am.

I think the most important point about being told something so huge and devastating is that it's very hard to take such news for real. It was very kind of you to tell us so soon after you knew and give us the chance to adjust to the idea. Though I can't say I am still fully present on the situation. It's so beyond anything I know. My way of dealing with most things is to keep trying and your health leaves me feeling that we simply must accept whatever happens.

In the beginning, right after you'd told us, I felt maybe nothing would really happen to you. I said to myself that there'd be a cure. I imagined the doctors were wrong. I went so far as to think or hope that you'd exaggerated. I told myself that you were always a dramatic person and that this fit neatly. Then I saw you again, a year later, and I had worked myself into such a state that I was disappointed you weren't transformed by the problem. I can't tell you who I imagined I would meet but I was angry that it was still you. (I think I wanted you to be a cause rather than a person.)

I hope you're laughing now at the absurdity of me being mad at you for being the you I was so terrified of losing. Perhaps this was a version of being mad at you for getting sick and threatening me with your absence. Whatever the explanation I can't say I was proud of my response.

I believe it was after that second visit that your father and I began to try to have a baby. That was a tricky decision. We didn't want to make ourselves unavailable to move to London if and when the need should arise. We also didn't know if you'd want us, or to be frank, if you would want me. The prospect of having an infant in America and your dad in England wasn't rosy. But we also couldn't put our lives on hold and grimly wait for the worst to happen to you.

I still somehow don't believe you're going to get AIDS. I just can't cope with the idea. And yet, every once in a while we'll hear a new statistic or read about a new drug or know someone who dies and your dad and I will look up at each other and cry in fear and worry for you.

Maybe we should have moved to London when you first told us. But then we would presume a priority in your life. We would need to have you respond to our ideas of how you should handle yourself. And you didn't ask us to take over your life. You're a grown woman. So we've gone on as usual, loving you, hoping that you won't develop AIDS, hoping that if you do get deathly ill that we can give you what you want and need and not what we want and need to give you. But knowing how imperfect life works itself out I doubt you're even happy now with what we're doing. We're all so defensive that we want to be in the right. That seems to be part of survival. And it seems ridiculous in the face of your being ill. Sad as it is, not knowing what's 'right' also makes it hard to know what to do or think about in your situation.

It took me more than a page, as you'd asked, but I took the liberty of writing more.

Love,

> *As ever,*
>> *Lucy*

PS: I consider this the beginning of a conversation. There is a lot I'd be happy to talk about. For instance your attitudes to drugs and to work and to the family.... But I will leave that to you to let me know that you want to hear more. You may not. I will understand either way.

In October 1989 I lost two close friends to AIDS. In the same month my father and Lucy's son Nicholas was born, just before the San Francisco earthquake, and exactly a quarter of a century after my first brother Mathew. I wonder how different life for him will be, growing up in that city in the 1990s? But his birth was, for me, a reminder that amidst the pain and the deaths and loss, life goes on.

When I look back I recognize that I've had a lot of chances that other people have not. In many ways life's been easy for me. I've had lucky breaks at the right times and good people around me. My family have, for the most part, been kind, long suffering and understanding. Often more supportive than I deserved. The same goes for my chosen family, my friends. Although with hindsight I might have done things differently, then again, maybe I wouldn't have. I have to believe we can take something from every experience - even our mistakes. That we can turn them around and use them to construct something better in our lives now. I have had the privilege of not having to remain silent. I was able to make that choice supported and protected by the people I am close to. Because of what AIDS has been made to represent, most women are not able to make that choice. Our voices are not heard. We live in isolation and fear of discovery. We remain invisible. Often people ask if I regret having been tested. I don't know. I can't imagine life without HIV now. It's become too much a part of who I am and how I lead my life. Even if I forget, it's always there, lurking, some place not too far from the surface. Whether my life untested would have been better or worse, I can't say. Different? Yes. For sure.

How has writing this has changed me? It's odd writing all this down because you don't remember things in words. It's mainly images and feelings and those I can't convey. It's been unsettling because as I think back and reflect on what happened, I remember other things that happened that change it all and change how I feel now. Shifting ground. There's a lot of anger too that I didn't realize was there or maybe just didn't allow myself to remember was there. There's also a lot of love and fondness and appreciation for people that I'd not recognized before.

But when I read it back it reads all wrong. It looks like somebody's story, not mine. That person isn't me. Imagined histories. Some here on paper, mine and those of some of the people close to me, others nowhere else but in our heads, re-writing the past in different ways. So who can prove or dis-prove what we remember? What makes it 'real'? And who can tell the difference? And in the end who cares? What matters to me is being here, now, and that I have a future to look forward to, whatever it may bring. But I'm not going to waste too much time thinking or worrying about it because if I do that I might just forget to enjoy what's happening right under my nose!

SUE

*Sue is in her mid-thirties; a registered
nurse and midwife. She became involved
in feminism in the early 1980s. She has
been living in the Midlands with HIV
since 1987.*

I NEVER KNEW until years later the real reason why all my
teachers supported my decision to become a naval nurse. They
thought that it would knock some sense into me. It didn't. I
lasted a month. It was a good month.

I think, for me, being a nurse gave me an identity. When I
was eleven years old I was removed abruptly from my mother's
home to live with my father. She had been given a choice. Lose
the husband who was sexually abusing her daughter or lose both
children. She chose the latter. I never thought much of that
decision. The problem was, that in removing me from sexual
danger, I was also removed from my friends and my roots. I
drifted in and out of school cliques; I never felt that I should
become close to anyone just in case the same thing happened
again. I also felt that in some way it was my fault that I was
abused. That I was available in some way. It wasn't until years
later that I could clarify these thoughts. If anyone had said in
my teenage years that I thought I was worthless I would have
laughed in their face.

So becoming a nurse seemed like a good idea at the time.
You know, the uniform, 'doctor's orders', the boarding school
atmosphere of the Nurses' Home. At about the same time I
commenced my sexual adventures.

The best description is to say that I was sexually indiscrimi-
nate. I dispute the word 'promiscuous'. It is not a word gen-

erally associated with sexually active men, so why women?

Anyway, to continue with the story, shortly after qualifying as a general nurse I started midwifery training. This was for no better reason than I had a year to kill before I was twenty-five years old (twenty-five was then the minimum age that nurses could work on P & O and Cunard liners). I had decided to return to the Navy. If not the Royal, then the Merchant Navy would do. As it happens, I ended up loving midwifery. Possibly it had something to do with the hospital where I trained. Or the theory that midwives were an autonomous body, able to work with other health professionals, not for them. After I qualified I moved to a city, started working in a large maternity hospital and continued with my sexual adventures.

I cannot say that all my sexual encounters were casual. I have had a few serious relationships. Unfortunately none of these lasted. I had become adept at wrecking any relationship which threatened to involve some commitment from me. This scenario repeated itself often. And although I destroyed these relationships, sometimes quite brutally, I never realized that I had continued a pattern which had started in my teens.

In the early 1980s I joined a women's group. This proved to be one of the best decisions of my life. I'll never forget the end of that meeting in that cold draughty hall. It was 6 May 1981. Everyone else pulled out their *Spare Rib* diary and I had a *Cosmopolitan* one. I was so embarrassed. I thought I wouldn't be admitted to 'their club' because I had failed a test. It was through this group that I started to understand a lot about myself.

While all this self-discovery was going on I was still working at the same maternity hospital. I started to challenge a lot of my own attitudes and prejudices and I began to criticize a lot of my colleagues' behaviour. The passive racist remarks like, 'I don't know why these Asian women complain about their treatment, I treat everyone the same,' grated. It was as if a curtain had been pulled from my eyes. I remember one senior midwife writing on the progress board about a woman, 'SHE SMOKES CANNABIS' in big red letters. Everybody read that board; cleaners, visitors, everyone. I began to realize how bigoted a lot of midwives were. It was an uphill struggle sometimes just keeping my mouth shut. I know that I wasn't very popular with some of my erstwhile colleagues. I can't really blame them. Tact was not my middle name.

One of my friends became pregnant. She was a lesbian. At about the time of delivery date I asked if I could deliver her baby. Permission refused. It would have been all right if she had been a 'normal heterosexual' woman I found out later. But because she was a lesbian it was decided that she had no right to choose her own midwife. If this sounds a bit paranoid I also found out that several of my colleagues had delivered their friends' babies over the years in the same hospital.

Eventually I started applying for different jobs. There were many reasons for this decision. Some personal, some professional. In late 1984 I left my promising career in the health service to work in Southern Africa. One of my reasons for choosing this particular job was to see if I was as anti-racist as I thought I was. In retrospect I can't think of a more foolish reason but, as they say, it seemed like a good idea at the time. I stayed in there for two years. There were some bad times. Common sense says there were, but the only two rough times that I can clearly remember are in 1986 when I was admitted to hospital with various dreadful ailments including mild jaundice and an incomplete miscarriage and in April 1987 when I was raped. In fact I don't remember the actual attack but the physical damage to my body left me in no doubt that the lift I had accepted from the white farmer had ended in disaster.

So I returned to England with various memories, a tan, a promise of marriage if I returned to Africa, Hepatitis B immune, bilharzia, and HIV positive.

I was tested for HIV antibodies during a routine end of contract medical examination. The story goes something like this: I told the doctor about my admission to hospital, contracting some kind of hepatitis, the sexually transmitted diseases I had caught (knowing why I went on the sexual merry-go-round hadn't stopped me from having the odd ride). He said to me, 'Do you want the HIV test?' I agreed. Now if that sounds a bit stark let me explain a bit. I had been working in a country where HIV and AIDS was becoming common. I knew about the risks I had been taking with my body, and if I was positive I wished to know about it straight away. It was the same when I had teeth removed, I always wanted to see the offending tooth.

Eventually, to cut another interesting tale short, I received my results. Over the phone, nine o'clock on a Monday morning, just after I had accepted a job in my local hospital. He really did not want to tell me that way, but when I told him that I would assume I was HIV positive unless he told me otherwise then he had no choice. He said that he was so sorry. That amused me. I mean unless he had something to do with me contracting the virus what had he to be sorry about?

To be honest, although I wasn't shocked by the result, in the back of my mind there had been some hope that the spectre had not sat down at my feast. I did all the right things in those first days of positive knowledge. I phoned various helplines. I listened to all this good advice, you know the sort of advice well-meaning people give, 'no sex', 'you'll have to eat well now', 'don't tell anyone else', 'there's no point in starting a new career, just be thankful you have a secure job'. I think that was the most ironic piece of advice that anyone gave me. Just going to work at that hospital caused stress. When you're on a diet the only adverts you ever take any notice of are the food ones. I found the same with being HIV positive. If there was any conversation around the subject I seemed to hear it, and it was usually all bad. A student nurse once voiced an opinion that if she was asked to look after 'an AIDS victim' she would resign first, after all she had her family to think of. All around me I saw nods of agreement. Nowadays when I give talks to health professionals there are murmurs of disapproval when I cite these examples. But I bet if I went into other hospital dining-rooms I would hear similar statements. I was so depressed. I only took the job to save money before I returned to marry the unwitting cause of my present predicament. Now I was trapped, seemingly forever, to have my ears assaulted with half truths about my own condition. I longed to be able to shout, 'You've got it all wrong. People like me don't have two heads. We're normal!' But of course we weren't. We had all done something wrong and now we were being punished.

For me the final straw was when I attended a midwives' refresher course. It was July 1988. I sat and listened to midwives stating openly that if they were at all unsure of a woman's background at the ante-natal booking clinic they would authorize the HIV test for that woman, without her knowledge or consent of course. After all, the midwives had a right to know. If there was a risk of infection the midwives had to protect themselves, didn't they? When I argued that I worked in a country where there was a high incidence of syphilis, and that we never handled any blood products of anyone without gloves, the vociferous delegates stated that there would be no need to do that if the woman's status was known. I had never come across such implacable self-righteousness before. I had always thought that a lot of my colleagues were rigid and unrealistic, but now it was as if they had no concept of people's individual rights as human beings. The tutors worked hard at changing attitudes but it was to no avail. I was stunned the whole week, and got through it in a drunken haze. And please don't ask if there was anyone at work in whom I could confide. There wasn't anyone there I could trust. Mind you there were plenty of people who would shout from the treetops 'AIDS VICTIM HERE!' Luckily, for my sanity, I broke down at a friend's house and they put me in touch with a local Body Positive group. Soon after I applied for, and was successful in obtaining, another job in a different city. The day I received the letter confirming the post I walked out of that hospital, determined never to enter its portals again.

The story does not end there however. I specifically did not tell my present employers about my status. There was no intention to deceive. But I felt that as long as I was fit and well my HIV status was my concern, not my employer's. I slowly rebuilt my life. I began to realize that although there was a downside to being positive, there was an upside too. I started to value my life, possibly for the first time since I was eleven years old. I contacted old friends and made new ones. I only accepted into my life people who were good for me. I also started to talk about my status openly. I built up a previously shattered existence into something worthwhile. Then, one day during a supervision session, my line manager disclosed that she had known about my HIV positive status ever since she had received my medical form from my previous doctor. Despite my verbal and written instructions to the contrary, he had recorded my status on the medical form. And he was too much of a coward to tell me. My employers had been in a quandary because they did not know if I knew of my status because of the way it had been disclosed to them. Eventually they decided to tell me of their knowledge when the situation seemed appropriate. I still work for the same organization.

So where am I at this moment in my life? I have a lover who is also a friend. We've been together for nearly two years now. I have a good job and loyal, true friends. I think I am very fortunate. I am still trying to make some sense out of all this. Occasionally I am still haunted by my past. I don't think of 'what if I wasn't positive?' Because in some strange way being positive has given me some meaning in my life. I have goals to achieve, mountains to climb, rivers to swim and people to love.

Writing this has been difficult. Not because I didn't want to share the information, but I didn't know how to. As with all personal stories there is often too much to tell. I had a problem deciding what to put in and what to leave out. There were so many avenues I could have travelled down with you. Also in writing about my so-called professional colleagues' attitudes about HIV and AIDS I wanted to share some personal feelings. I have so much more to tell. So many adventures to share and so many still to come. The story has not ended here.

VIV

*Viv was born in 1960 and now lives alone
in London with her cats. She enjoys
travelling, eating and shopping. She was
diagnosed HIV positive in 1991.*

I WAS BORN in the West Country and came to London to work
ten years ago. I have recently celebrated my thirty-second
birthday. I went for a test in March of 1991, thinking that there
was no way in the world that I would be positive. I wasn't part
of a so-called 'high risk' group as far as I knew. You tend to
think that if you're not a drug user yourself, and if you only
have a few boyfriends all of whom you know well, none of
whom were bisexual or gay, then you must be okay. You think
you've had no contact with any 'high risk' groups and aren't
in one yourself, so there's no problem. When I went back for
the result the doctor said, 'Bad news!'

I've gone over it so many times now, how did I manage to
pick up the virus? It must have been through sex. Although I
put it down to one particular boyfriend, possibly I'm being
unfair. I haven't heard anything from that guy. I know now
that he was a drug user, so I've linked the two things together,
but that's a bit of a stereotype.

I sent a letter saying I was HIV positive to another boy I
met last year, but he didn't get back to me. I've got friends
who live in the same town in Italy, and I got them to go and
see him, to make sure he was all right. It must be shattering
news to get a letter like that. It would blow your mind.
Apparently he took my letter to his doctor and the doctor told
him he was a perfectly healthy and strong person and therefore he couldn't have picked up the virus from me. And then

he said that even if he had picked it up he would have shown some signs of illness by now! I'm going to visit Italy soon, and I'm thinking about going along to this doctor and saying 'Find something wrong with me, jerk!'

I went for a test because I've got a group of friends in Germany who I've known for years and they are very into the idea that it's responsible to have an HIV test. A couple of them had had the test and it had come back negative. Perhaps the greatest motivation for me was seeing a German friend last year. She wasn't a very close friend, but we always kept in touch. The last time I saw her she looked fine, just very tired. Then I heard she had been taken into hospital with full-blown AIDS and had only a short time to live. She had a boyfriend who had to have an HIV test to come to live with her in Germany. At that time he was HIV negative but a year and a half after living with her he was positive. All that made me think about the virus seriously and I decided to have the test to set my mind at ease.

I had counselling before I had the test done. I remember that my doctor was very nice, he was really upset having to tell me the news. But I was in so much shock, I was knocked for six! He kept saying that I was taking it so well, maybe I'd suspected I had it already. But of course I hadn't. I had this strange experience of shaking inside, underneath my skin. I had to wait a while before seeing a counsellor and there were a couple of guys who had probably come for the test too, but they didn't look as if they had received bad news, so I sat there thinking I had to stay in control or the guys would guess. Maybe it would have been good if I'd been able to talk to them, they probably would have given me a shoulder to cry on.

I went back to work after the result and for about an hour or two I carried on normally. I went out and did some shopping and suddenly all I could think of was getting home as quickly as possible. The next day I took off from work and then it was the weekend and then I took a week to go to Germany. That was wonderful. My friend there is into homeopathic and alternative medicine and took me to see a doctor there. I couldn't see the point at first, after all he was in Germany. But I went along and he was really, really nice and very positive, which was different from the English doctor. He told me I had to try and remain positive, eat well and stay healthy. He told me stories of people who had the virus for as long as fifteen years or so. He spent about an hour and a half talking with me. He was an alternative doctor and he said there was no point in giving me any medicine because I was well. He gave me an immune modulator, a blood purifier, which in Germany is quite a common thing to take.

Very recently my T-cell count has gone down and that's been a bit depressing. I'm still very healthy but the count is down. My doctor here says that the T-cell count is only a marker, and as I'm still very healthy I don't want to get obsessed with the meaning of that count. I keep taking the immune modulators and I also take all sorts of vitamins. The advice about vitamins is confusing because even the alternative practitioners differ: some say take a lot and others say don't, you might harm yourself. Deciding how much to take is a difficult decision. My doctor mentioned AZT but I really don't know whether to take it or not. I don't really want to take it, but if I have to, I will. I'm chicken and I'll take anything when it comes down to it.

I go to an alternative health clinic in London. I very rarely take any chemicals. It's easy to say that but when you start analyzing the things you eat or drink, right away you're looking at food colourings, for instance. As far as medicines are concerned I don't take anything. I'm lucky because I'm well, but I don't even take aspirins. I believe there is a lot of power in the brain, which is why I try to do visualization.

My friends were all very shocked when I told them I was positive. I didn't tell them face to face which was a good thing in my case. It's very traumatic to tell someone that way. I told most people over the phone. Luckily everyone said 'Hi, how are you?' Then it was my turn to say, 'Oh, all right for somebody who's just found out they're HIV positive.' Work caused me a lot of problems because everyone said you shouldn't tell people at work, or at least think very, very carefully about it. So I thought, and it was really getting me down because it was such a strain having to lie about where you were going when you had a hospital appointment. You can't predict how long an appointment will take and you have to wait. So I decided to go to see our accountant and I told him and asked him if he thought I should tell my colleagues. We decided they would take the news all right, so he phoned them up and on some pretext said we all needed to meet in his office. I told them all there. It was traumatic and one colleague said it was the only time she had been made speechless in her whole life. Another colleague knew quite a lot on the subject which was good. On the whole, for me, it was the right thing to have done.

I almost didn't get in touch with Positively Women. I came away from getting my result with an idea that if you went to a support group, you'd see people who were really ill and that would be depressing and end up harming you. I knew Kate from Positively Women a bit from ages ago. We have a mutual friend and I met her at parties which is ironic because years ago this mutual friend told me he knew a girl who was HIV positive and that it wasn't easy for her because most of the groups she went to were all men. I remember having this conversation at a dinner party where we were talking about using condoms and a couple of people were saying they always used them and me and another girl were wondering aloud about what happens if you're really drunk, do you always use them then?

Another friend of Kate's gave me Positively Women's number. I called after I had the news of my T-cell count. I'd gone to Covent Garden and bought this big fluffy jumper as a consolation prize. I went for something to eat and I was getting more and more tearful. In the restaurant there was a family with children and I couldn't bear seeing happy people at that moment. So I went round the corner and called Positively Women. I'm so glad I did because it has made such a difference, being able to go to small groups with other positive women. It's such a beautiful building, very calm and peaceful, like a haven.

RITA

*Rita is a thirty-five-year-old African
woman who has lived in London for
three years.*

I CAME TO this country from Africa for political reasons. I
was diagnosed HIV antibody positive in May of the same year
when I was thirty-four years old. My father was a politician
and because of his political beliefs he was killed and my family
tortured. There are many people here because of political repression at home, but now, because I'm not very well, I don't
associate with any political groups.

At home I worked hard for many years in a good professional
job. When I came to England, I was forced to leave my children
with my mother. I miss them very much. At home I lived with
my mother and children five miles out of town and we had someone to look after the children while I was out at work. My
children still expect to join me here, but I have a problem about
their visas.

I stayed with some of my family who live here when I first
arrived. Quite soon after that I started getting swollen glands
and feet. I think they started suspecting me before I did myself, because they all knew about the AIDS epidemic in my
country. But I didn't know anything. I got a rash on my back
and went to the GP who gave me some antibiotics which didn't
help at all. My GP then advised me to go for further tests but
I left it for a while, because I didn't think there was anything
seriously wrong. Finally I was referred to a hospital where I
was given an HIV test which came back positive.

I never told my family here; I was scared I'd be sent away.
Eventually I had to leave anyway. They had stopped me from

131

using the washing machine and other household things, so it was clear that even though I didn't tell them, they suspected. People are still ignorant about the virus and in need of more education. Now I ring my family sometimes. I even brought my sister-in-law to see where I live, but we never talk about AIDS, we just talk about other things.

Everything was so hard. I contacted my social worker and through her I was given this flat. It was my social worker who also put me in contact with Positively Women. When I had the test, the people at the hospital were sympathetic and spent time talking to me, but I can't even remember what they said, because it was such a shock. By then I had no friends of my own at all, nobody to talk to. I spent about five months without sleeping because I didn't know what to do or where to go. I thought I was going to die. When I found out about Positively Women, it was the first group I went to, and I started going there almost everyday. Then I didn't feel so hopeless because I met so many women. A good thing about Positively Women is that many of the women working there are positive themselves. After that I knew I wasn't the only person with the virus and I also met other Africans who I would never have known otherwise.

My husband and I split up three years before I came to England, but I know he is all right. I must have got the virus from the boyfriend I was with after him. There is not enough education about HIV at home; some people are even scared of using condoms. They think they might get infected from them. The first time my boyfriend and I made love, I persuaded him to put on a condom, but he made a hole in it. I didn't know this because I was not the one who put it on. When we made love, I realized the condom was on but there was a very big hole in it, and I realized he had tricked me. Men think they won't get the feeling they do when they go without a condom.

Since I was diagnosed, I always get my boyfriend to use condoms. But I've had boyfriends who don't like to use them. They say no, no, I trust you. I told my boyfriend I was HIV positive but I think he believes I'm joking. Some time ago I told another man I was positive and he disappeared, he never came back to me again. That made me scared of telling anyone else, but of course I had to. He didn't disappear but I know he thinks I'm joking somehow. Sometimes he says he doesn't want to use condoms because he wants a child. As far as making love goes, men from home only know sexual intercourse. They don't know other ways of making love. They can romance, but they don't think it's enough, and I think many women feel the same way.

I go to Positively Women support group every Thursday and then to another one during the week at Landmark. Right now I'm feeling all right, but I still like going to a lot of groups. I meet friends and we exchange news. We talk about ourselves, how we feel, especially when we are unwell. You meet positive people who are happy. I've had bronchitis and in 1991 I got shingles. Those things made my immune system weaker, so these days I'm tired all the time and feel very weak. I took AZT for three weeks but then I stopped it for the time being because it made me feel worse: I lost my appetite, I was vomiting and had diarrhoea. Now, except for the tiredness I'm okay. I inhale Pentamidine which helps to prevent PCP, once every month. I talked to someone at Positively Women about my diet and she advised me to eat things like high fibre food and brown rice which are good for my health. I take kelp powder which tastes terrible but is supposed to help my immune system. Also I often get a massage from someone at London Lighthouse or at the Landmark which is very good. I like acupuncture; I find it painful but it helps.

I'm much less scared now that I'm going to die. I hope I will live until there's a solution. When I talk to people at Positively Women who have been positive for years, it makes me feel that I'll still live for some years to come.

At the moment I'm not doing anything. I would love to have a baby if I had a job, but there's no way now that I could look after a baby. If my children were able to join me I would have to leave this flat because it wouldn't be big enough. The housing association this flat is part of only houses single women, so I would have to find another place. I get social security and I'm entitled to the disabled premium but I still wish I could work because I'm not used to sitting at home all the time, and I think doing nothing makes me feel tired. I try to go to a gym and go swimming. Sometimes I see people in the evening, especially if I go to a group, but other times I go to bed early.

Even if I was able to work, it would be risky because some people don't want to hire a person with the virus. There are people who still think they can catch it from a cup. Three friends I had are scared of being seen with me and can't even bring themselves to say hello; they pass by as if they haven't seen me, as if they don't know me. They've heard the rumour that I'm HIV positive.

When I was first tested I cried a lot and even felt ashamed. One of my friends rang home and said I was dying, so my ex-husband rang up to find out what was happening and what I was dying of. I told him I wasn't sick at all, but he started suspecting. My children don't know yet. Sometimes I get angry, especially when I am very lonely. Even if you have a special friend in this country you can never see him every day. Life is so different here; everyone has their own problems and lives so far apart. If I had my children I know I could be happy making them a home.

Positively Women is important because I know I can say whatever I want and I can talk to people who are like me. It's better that we're all women together. An African group has begun meeting and that is going to be a regular thing. I don't really know if we need a special group for black women since everyone there is positive. I haven't made up my mind yet. I know that going to Positively Women took away some of my fears and loneliness. There are other women the same as me, we can share things and give each other confidence.

PEARL

Pearl is a lecturer on women and children with HIV/AIDS. She is a thirty-seven-year-old mother of one child and two cats and is a former director of Positively Women. She is HIV positive.

GROWING UP ON a farm which was really part of Cape Town in South Africa was idyllic in many ways except that my parents got divorced when I was young. As a child I found my mum a vital woman but quite selfish, and I didn't get on well with her. It wasn't until recently that I could look back and accept her for herself. At the time she seemed impossibly glamorous and removed.

I loathed my Catholic schooling; I experienced the hypocrisy and strict catholicism of the nuns at a very young age. We weren't Catholics, so the only reason my parents sent me there was because it was meant to be a good girls' school. In those days parents didn't worry about a girls' education because the expectation was that you would get married and be looked after. My brother was the one whose education was deemed important. Academically my school was appalling but they turned out 'nice young ladies', which was a joke because by the time we left most of us were well into drugs or had been pregnant.

I had a political awareness from a young age which was probably brought about by my schooling. We were told that all people were equal in the eyes of God so I would ask why there were only white children at the school? It was my experiences as a child which made me question. I grew up on a farm with 'coloured' and black children, then they were systematically excluded from my school, and as we grew older even playing together was frowned upon. I knew there was something wrong underneath it all.

Socially and culturally, compared to Britain, South Africa was still like the 1950s for the white population. Abortion was illegal and completely unacceptable socially. Yet there was a youth counter-culture which was influenced by what was happening in the West. At about fourteen I'd started smoking dope and was hanging around with hippies and people involved in the peace movement, as well as with surfers who came from all over the world. They brought in a lot of music and magazines from other countries which were banned in South Africa; everything was banned or censored. For me another side to these involvements was contact with black South Africans. This happened through the music we were all crazy about and smoking dope. These racially mixed gatherings were seen as political although I don't think many of us defined them for ourselves as political. There were illegal gigs, where we'd just get together and have a wonderful time. But we'd have to have lookouts so we'd be able to get away if the police arrived.

When I was sixteen in 1970 I got pregnant. It was an extremely traumatic experience. I didn't tell anyone until I was seven months along and couldn't squeeze into my school uniform any longer. I was too terrified to tell my mother but when I did she said if I'd come to her earlier she could have taken me to Mozambique where abortion was legal. There was no option, it wasn't the done thing to be a young unmarried mother, and so she took me up to Zululand and I went through the farce of pretending to be married while I waited for the birth. I knew nothing about pregnancy let alone labour. I had no check-ups. When I went into labour I was totally shocked but I lay there on my back and gave birth to a daughter who was taken away from me immediately. There was no choice; I was told either I got married or the baby was adopted, that's it! When we got back to Cape Town my mother told everyone I'd had glandular fever and I never talked to anyone about what had happened.

After that I refused to return to school. My mother's response was that if I wasn't going to school I had to go to work. From the year after having the baby until I came to London, I went completely loopy. Perhaps it was a nervous breakdown although I certainly didn't realize it at the time. I was heavily into politics which involved putting myself at risk from the authorities. I didn't do many drugs, just smoked a bit of dope, but my mental state was all over the place. Finally my grandmother, whom I'd always adored and who always talked to me about being independent and having my own life, talked to me about her concern that I might be arrested soon and suggested that I leave the country. She gave me the money and I booked my passage to England. I left when I was just eighteen.

I arrived in England straight from a very hot summer in South Africa into the middle of an intensely cold winter. Everything seemed so big, the numbers of people, the size of the city, but at the same time it seemed grey, ugly, and dirty. It was total culture shock. Luckily I met an amazing woman who quickly took me under her wing and helped to settle me into a large hippie house in Notting Hill Gate. There was a real mixture of people living in the house and I felt great there. A Scottish poet who visited said we were all playing at poverty and I suppose we were. But it was just what I needed, the best thing that could have happened to me at that point. I also met a guy who informed me he was gay or bisexual but at the time I didn't understand what that meant. We fell in love, he moved in with me and without much reflection we got married. I remember it as being a sunny, happy period. Perhaps for me it was like a liberation because for the first time ever I could say whatever I wanted to and not worry about being arrested.

After three years Tim and I had an untraumatic split up, basically because we realized we were best friends, not lovers. We hadn't slept together for ages and at the age of twenty-one, much as we loved each other, there wasn't much point in staying together. Anyway, by that point, I think he was pining for boys.

When I was in South Africa we didn't have any television, but the one thing you could get hold of and listen to was music and fantastic radio stations from Mozambique and other places. Quite by accident in London I met a couple of songwriters who were impressed with my knowledge of music. One of them rang me up to say he'd got me an interview to work on The Who management team. I got the job. God knows why they hired me as I hadn't a clue about working a switchboard or much else. I found myself working in the rock and roll business. At first I was a receptionist but because there were so few of us working there, I ended up doing whatever needed doing and learned on the job about things like tours, concerts, publicity, the whole business of bringing out records. It was busy and very good; a big learning process.

I moved to a flat in Notting Hill, on my own for the first time. The music scene changed, punk came in and I changed along with it. By now things were running so smoothly in my job that I felt the urge to move on - I wanted to learn more about working in music at the grass roots level. I went to work for another management group who looked after up and coming bands, controversial groups who didn't have any money and were struggling. Finally I started getting into making music videos with a bunch of friends who worked in film. It started off more as a joke; we got £2,000 to do two videos which we thought was a fortune, but then it really took off as big business. Suddenly there were a handful of us who were known as the experts, getting huge budgets and big bands to feature.

My daughter's dad moved in with me from the first night we went out. We started travelling around the world a lot - to the Caribbean, the USA, all over. When I first met him he was a graphic and comic artist who wanted to get into the work I was doing for a set designer. We landed up working together, doing art direction and soon he started directing and producing. I fell pregnant just as he started to direct. We decided to get married and I realized that of course Tim and I were still married. It was all resolved easily because Tim had moved in to share the flat with us and we were all friends. We got a quickie divorce and I married S when I was eight months pregnant with Tim as our best man. When I went into labour S went rushing in and woke Tim up and we all went to the hospital together. When they asked who the husband was they both answered 'I am'. We couldn't stop laughing.

After my child was born in 1983, S and I started having big problems. He was doing a lot of coke, working extremely long hours in a situation where for the first time I wasn't working with him. There were probably resentments on both sides and we didn't put them right. When my daughter was about two and half months old, S was doing a job in Los Angeles and wanted me to join him there. I was breast-feeding and was reluctant to go but decided if I wanted to help make the relationship work I had to. I weaned the baby very quickly which was quite distressing and a girlfriend of mine looked after her while I was away. We went to Hawaii for a so-called honeymoon, but it wasn't working. We were on two different wavelengths. When we got back about a week later he got a job which took him to New York and this time I absolutely refused, I couldn't leave the baby.

While he was in New York he had a brief affair. I knew it immediately, instinctively - up until then we'd been completely faithful to each other. First of all he lied and swore he hadn't had an affair and that I was mad. He went back to New York still saying that nothing had happened. But a friend of mine there, with whom S was supposedly staying, got fed up with the situation and decided I should know the truth. My first reaction was relief that I knew the truth and that I wasn't mad. But then I went to pieces.

I decided to leave England with my baby and start a new life in Australia where my parents now lived. Everything felt in crisis; I'd lost a lot of weight, I was totally run down and all over the place. There was no work for me in Melbourne and I desperately needed work. Friends came through yet again; a film director in Sydney introduced me to film and video people there. I moved, found a flat and started the process of getting my life together again. S kept calling me, wanting us to get back together and when he came over at Christmas to see his daughter, he persuaded me to start over with him in Australia. I know it sounds crazy but against my better judgment, I did. And then he did the whole thing all over again!

Classic! We were working together again on an Elton John shoot I was producing when one night he never came home - and I knew, I just knew he was with someone else. I came on to the set in the morning, he wasn't there, and for him to be late was really unusual. Eventually he walked in with the video's principal dancer and she had his coat on. I only thought how dare he do this to me at work, on a big shoot, and of course he denied it. I'll never forget that day, trying to keep up appearances, trying to keep the shoot together, and really, I wanted to kill him. This time round I didn't have friends around and I wasn't 'at home' in Australia. At least before in England, I'd had wonderful girlfriends who literally moved in with me and didn't leave me alone for a minute. Not having any of that made it a hundred times worse.

There were a few friends, not so close, including two gay guys, who were very sweet. The two guys suggested we all go away for a few days. One of them had to go back to town and that night the two of us got absolutely wrecked. We were drunk, we had some mescaline, some coke, we went for it and we landed up sleeping together. I didn't think much about it at the time. I knew the two men weren't faithful to each other and sleeping with him made me feel better. It was the first time I'd been able to let go after S and I had our final split. Looking back, it's obvious that's where I got the virus. Funnily enough, at the time the guy's boyfriend was complaining of having a weird rash but of course it meant nothing very significant to us then.

Shortly after that experience I moved back to London. I had a baby, no home, and no money, but again my girlfriends and the couple I'd worked with who managed The Who, pulled me through. A girlfriend who had a baby the same age as mine and who was also a video producer needed a place to live and Tim was around looking for some place. So the three of us and the babies got a big house together in London. It turned into a very happy time - the two children adored each other and we all shared housework and childcare. Jackie and I started producing again and I got my life back onto an even keel - things were happening again.

I got diagnosed by accident. I had an abnormal cervical smear and was told I needed treatment for my cervix. But I continued to feel run down and not quite right - I knew something else was wrong. I went for a check-up from my doctor but a locum was there who got quite enthusiastic about finding out the cause of it all; he thought it might be glandular fever and took blood tests to find out. A few days later when the results were back he told me it wasn't that, so he'd requested an HIV test. I was furious and wanted him to stop it but it was too late, it was at the lab. In that case I didn't want to know the results, but I had a strong feeling that I was positive. By that time I knew a lot more about HIV and AIDS because I had a lot of gay friends and Tim worked as a journalist reporting on AIDS issues.

Two weeks later my own doctor turned up on my doorstep. As he'd never dropped in socially before, I knew what was coming. Although he knew I didn't want to know the results, he thought I must know that I was positive. Even though I'd suspected, being told for certain was a huge shock. My first reaction was wanting to know how much time I had left. Tim was there and the irony of it all struck both of us - there he was, a promiscuous gay man who for many pre-AIDS years had had unsafe sex, and his test had been negative. But my main fears were for my child. I was terrified she might be infected. It wasn't rational; I knew I got the virus after she was born. There wasn't as much knowledge around about transmission as there is now and I had visions of when she'd used my toothbrush, when she'd helped me clean up blood after I cut my finger.

These images rushed through my brain. And then I was concerned about my new partner, G. We'd been together for a few months, although we weren't living together, and we had an active unprotected sex life. He's got to be positive, I thought. The burden of breaking the news to him was frightening. I just couldn't face it. Tim said he'd do it for me and got him to come over while I went to wait at a girlfriend's. I waited and chain-smoked and jumped every time the phone went. When he finally rang he told me very gently and nicely to come on home. I remember driving back, how I don't know, I was shaking and crying so, but when I got there he put his arms around me and said he was relieved it was only HIV. We made love and I knew he wasn't going to reject me. I don't think it had really sunk in but it was a good reaction and it made a big difference to me.

After that, though, I began to feel very isolated. My doctor suggested I see a woman at his practice who turned out to be a wonderful person but she didn't know of any other women who were positive and she had no knowledge of specialist centres or voluntary support organizations. It was as if there was a sheet of glass between me and the rest of the world. I couldn't relate properly, other than to a few good friends. I wasn't rejected in any form or fashion but I did notice an uneasiness. In a way it was too close to home for many of my friends, because my behaviour had been no different from theirs - especially coming out of the music and television world where there was a lot of casual drug use and a lot of sleeping around among film crews. They didn't really want to take in the fact that I was positive, because if I was it wasn't out of the realm of possibilities that they could be. If I tried to talk about it there was definitely a feeling of discomfort - they didn't know how to cope with it.

Soon afterwards a close friend of mine, an actor living in New York who was HIV positive, came down with PCP. He was a vital, good looking man and very vain, very funny and it all hit him very hard. There were no preventative treatment then so he started losing weight quickly and losing his looks.

He didn't want to go into hospital so he asked Tim and me and a couple of other friends if we'd look after him, which turned out to be quite difficult for me to do. In a way it was like looking in a mirror of my worst fears.

My new boyfriend, G, lived in Norfolk and was married. He and his wife had some kind of open relationship which I didn't want to know about. It was all too complicated and confused for me to deal with. He didn't like me setting down any conditions or constraints but every time I sent him away to figure things out, he'd be back.

Nineteen-eighty-six was a traumatic year. I needed G, but on the other hand I didn't want our relationship the way it was. My actor friend died just before Christmas and G agreed that it was best if we stopped seeing each other while he and his wife tried to sort out whatever it was they wanted to do with their lives. Morbid thoughts kept coming into my mind. Would I be around next Christmas? What the hell was going to happen? As the final straw, I got the flu the day before New Year's Eve. It was the first illness I'd had since being diagnosed and even though it was only the flu it was terrible to go through because of course I feared it was much more than that.

A few days after New Year's when I was feeling a bit better, I got a call from a girl I'd known when I first came to this country who told me she was doing work with the Terrence Higgins Trust. She and a guy called Tony Whitehead and his boyfriend George wanted to put together a concert. Would I organize it? I was feeling isolated, so this suggestion was amazing; it immediately gave me something motivating to take hold of. The concert had to be held on the first of April somewhere like Wembley Stadium which gave me three months to pull it off. I thought, hell, that's an enormous amount of work for no money - and went ahead. Tony and George were great but they had no idea at all how to organize it so I was really on my own. I asked a girlfriend from the music and film video business to help. She knew all about my diagnosis and was more than pleased to help. We were given offices by the Marquee. The

whole thing was shambolic. But we had incredibly good vol-
unteers from all walks of life and everyone worked incredibly
hard. For the first time it hit me that there were other people
out there who weren't necessarily positive but who were affected by HIV and wanted to do something about the crisis.

Going round to music managers and musicians was something
else! All the managers and record company people didn't want
their artists to go anywhere near it because it was AIDS. The
press were printing gay plague stories and working up an anti-
gay backlash. George Michael was the first one to say he'd
do it which was brave because there were so many rumours
going round about him being gay. He stuck his neck out right
at the start, getting on to other musicians and people in the
business. Right up until almost the concert itself there was a
reluctance on the part of performers to appear, but about two
weeks before the date, the tide turned and we ended up with
more bands than we knew what to do with. Suddenly it got
trendy. We couldn't put them all on at Wembley so we got
lots of other venues in London in order not to waste the bands
who wanted to participate. We put on a whole week of events
and it spread right through all the major cities up to Scotland.
Wembley itself was something special. There were people who
cared and I know it made a lot of difference to people who were
positive or had AIDS. That experience empowered me and gave
me a lot of strength, but I still hadn't met any positive women.
There was nothing being done for women as far as I could see
and it was beginning to really bug me.

Because of the confidence I gained, after the concert I tried
to go back into mainstream work. At the time the Beastie Boys
were popular. Gilly, who did the concert with me, and I had
this silly idea to form a band and call it the Ghastly Girls. So
we got together three girls who were good singers and made a
band up. They told outrageous lies to the press and made up
truly ghastly stories about themselves. Gilly and I called ourselves Ghastly and Ghastly Management. We had a lot of good
fun with it but we couldn't believe how seriously we were

taken. Polly Toynbee came along to interview us and the girls - a whole page of the *Guardian* and it was all lies, complete lies. Everyone fell for it. We did one concert before there was even any music out and at one point we had front pages on newspapers, Sunday papers, and centre spreads. We got the band into a studio and as they were really very good musicians, the demos were out quickly. The joke was ours, but it began to turn sour when the girls started taking themselves seriously.

Not surprisingly I began thinking about doing something more relevant again. Thoughts about the virus were catching up with me, so when I was in the Terrence Higgins Trust one day, I asked if anyone there knew of any other positive women. Judy, who worked at the Trust said she thought there was an organization called Positively Women. She gave me a number and I remember calling and calling and getting an answerphone. Eventually Sheila rang and said there was a support group that Thursday. I was nervous about meeting other women after all this time. When I walked in Kate was there, although I missed meeting Sheila. Kate was the first one I met and we hit it off straight away and when I met Sheila a few days later we hit it off too. I felt as if I'd come home and I plunged right into the organization. There was so much work to do and I didn't want other women to go through the isolation I had. We had to let women know we existed. We were getting posters out and in to all the clinics and every women's organization we could think of. Fiona, who is presently our fundraiser, was then working as a temp in a charity and she used their computers to get our material out as well as trying to get us some funding in her spare time. With the first bit of money we got, we brought Fiona in full-time. That left me and the others more available to go out and do talks, as well as doing counselling and running a support group. Kate came in whenever she could but she was studying. Sheila was having some time off after the birth of her daughter which was also when she had her first bout of PCP. Even when Kate gave up her studies and came in full-time and Sheila was back the workload was intense with us all jammed into our tiny Kings Cross office. And we had more and more women coming in.

Working at Positively Women was an extremely empowering experience in such a different field for me. From entertainment, I was now working in the AIDS field with all women. All of us wanted to know every development around HIV and AIDS, we soaked up information, not just from here but from all over the world. I started getting more interested in the political side of the issue which brought me back to my younger South African self. Everything began to fit into place, almost as if all the experiences I'd had in the past were now coming in useful.

Personally I wasn't interested in relationships or sex during this time. I had one fling with a lovely guy in New York who was wonderful when I told him I was positive, but I wasn't in love with him and I wanted to get back to Positively Women. It also made me realize I wasn't over G yet. It's hard to believe but G called me when I got back from New York to say that he and his wife had split up. He wasn't over me either and we started up again.

At that time it was so chaotic at Positively Women that I really couldn't spare much time from it and I ended up feeling pulled in all directions. I was totally overloaded. There were arguments and problems between those of us in the office which coincided with the first women who were using our services becoming really ill. And finally we had our first death. I was doing a lot of hospital visits and finding them stressful but there wasn't any way for me to get support. I didn't want to burden my co-workers because they were going through similar things. My health started to suffer, I had blackouts, couldn't stop shaking. I was exhausted but through it all I kept it away from G who was still living in Norfolk. It isn't surprising that the everything caught up with me.

After a short holiday, I decided to hand in my resignation to Positively Women, a decision I felt strange about but it was necessary for me. By now there were six full-time staff, management was in place, we'd got new premises and were only waiting to move in, so I didn't feel I was letting anyone down. I was still committed to doing talks, and World AIDS Day 1990 was coming up and would be focused on the issue of women and AIDS. I was already set up to do quite a lot of television work which I intended to carry through. By Christmas I cut off.

I had developed a strong craving to go back to South Africa to see my mum and the country. My feelings about the virus were changing again. When I was at Positively Women, I was constantly working for other women, and it was as if I were partially in denial about my own status. It's difficult to describe, but suddenly I was becoming more aware of my personal virus. I certainly didn't want to die whenever, and not without going home first. G picked up on my state of mind and suggested he and his son and my daughter and I all go together. We went for about two months, a strange time as it happened to coincide with the Gulf War. The country has changed, many exiles were returning and there was a fantastic atmosphere. After forty years of repression and not being allowed to talk to each other, suddenly people had verbal diarrhoea. Irrespective of what colour you were, or what age, everyone was talking about the new South Africa and how to make it work.

I decided not to tell my mother about the virus because she has cancer and was struggling to survive herself. But she knew all about the work I'd been doing and had seen a few magazine articles about AIDS so I was able to talk about it in a general way. My stepsister was a matron in a hospital and I'd spoken to her about AIDS a number of times. One time when she was meant to be coming to dinner, she rang to say she couldn't make it because they had just had their first AIDS patient admitted, and everyone was busy disinfecting the room and so on. It was part of my realization of how backward South Africa was in relation to AIDS and what a serious absence of information and knowledge there was.

G was in the process of falling in love with South Africa

and deciding we should all live there. I decided to track down Body Positive in Cape Town, where I found only two guys, one of them very ill. It was the usual story: no women, no drugs available at all, no support. Homosexuality is still illegal (though in Cape Town especially, which is quite a gay city, no one ever took any notice), but it meant gay groups couldn't get registered as charities and receive funds. One of the guys was about to set off to New York or San Francisco to buy drugs to bring back and keep in his own fridge - he knew a couple of gay doctors who would administer them for him. Basically the South African government saw AIDS as a problem for drug users, gay men, and black people, all of whom they didn't think were worth much effort. It was more like Britain years ago but with no treatment available. It was so depressing and it made me realize I couldn't live there. I tried to explain it all to G but he couldn't understand. He couldn't grasp why I would need any support, or why I needed to know there were treatments available if I needed them.

It dawned on me that he hadn't really taken in my situation fully; he had been in some sort of denial for most of the time we were together. He never came to the hospital with me and didn't go through any of the deaths. I had contributed to his denial by keeping as much as possible away from him. As long as I seemed healthy and strong it didn't enter his head what it was really all about. Not surprisingly we ended up having a big argument, during which many things came to the surface. After that I felt conflicting emotions; here he was saying he'd finally made a commitment to me and why was I creating problems. I exploded, I felt I was coming out of a pod: this is me, I'll live my life the way I want to! He left the next day and I stayed on for a week to go and see my mum again. She couldn't understand what had happened and of course I couldn't explain the whole story fully. When my daughter and I returned to London, G and I tried to talk it out again - he was in a state of shock and simply couldn't understand why I was behaving as I was. I tried, he tried, but it didn't work and that was the end for us.

Since then I've started working again and I've benefitted from an excellent counsellor with whom I've been able to work through a lot. I do many of my talks through Positively Women and although I'm not working for them, I'm always aware of the need to advertise their existence. Most of the talks I do are for hospitals, doctors, nurses and social workers and I've done a few for children's homes. I'm really busy now, but in a way which isn't so stressful for me. It's not so emotional, and I've realized some important things. One is that I cannot work with any restrictions around me and will eventually rebel if they exist. Positively Women became too big for me and ended up strangling me. Too much time was spent in management meetings, or writing reports and I work better spontaneously.

I've always said my girlfriends were there, it doesn't matter what we've been through, we've always been there for each other. I needed that security within the context of HIV/AIDS and I've found that most other positive women need it too. Even if you have to go back to an existence where nobody knows about the virus, the fact you know your support group exists, comforts you. It really didn't matter what age, profession, culture, spiritual belief, or sexuality you were. Once together, we found that underneath so much is the same: emotions, problems with relationships, security, fears, hopes. Whether someone was heterosexual or lesbian, we still were able to discuss things together. I could talk about the need I have to give my daughter a crash course in life because most of the mums in Positively Women felt the same way. If none of us were positive we might have been able to talk about these things in other kinds of groupings, but unfortunately the virus is what makes us different from (and to) other women so we need to give each other support.

Since coming back from South Africa, I've recognized that a bit of me was tempted to have a so-called 'normal life', to get married, settle down. But I'm not normal in that respect and what happened between me and G in South Africa finally made me face up to the fact that for me it was all a fantasy. It doesn't work for me. Since then I've really wanted my child to have as much knowledge as possible, never to have it indoctrinated into her, as happened to me and so many women I know, that the only ideal is to have a family and a steady husband. I want her to know that life isn't necessarily like that, that it's incredibly flexible, that satisfaction and happiness don't have to be attached to one vision.

Thinking back to Positively Women, probably what women like Kate, Sheila and I have in common is that we're not afraid to speak out, so we take on the role of speaking on behalf of others and it becomes almost like a duty. If very few others are going to do it, then other women are relying on us to tell their stories, to get recognition and funding. Sometimes at Positively Women we would spot other women who had the potential to take on responsibility and try to encourage them to take on similar roles to ours. We really wanted some of the pressure to be eased, but often they either realized the pressure would be too much or they got involved, but not as spokeswomen.

Positively Women has helped women living with HIV to set up groups in other parts of the UK, but one of the problems is that if there's a support group in a small area, you may end up advertising your status. People will know it's run by positive women for positive women. I suppose you might get a local health authority in a small community to give you a room somewhere where support group meeting could be advertised - but there is still a reluctance and the smaller the community the more chance there is of being found out. I come across it even in London. I haven't told my child my status yet, although she's very up on HIV and AIDS. She surprised me a couple of weeks ago when I took her on the march at the end of the Reach Out and Touch conference in London. She wasn't altogether happy about going on it and asked me why she had to. I explained that it was for people who have already died of AIDS and for those who are living with HIV - to show that we care. Then she asked me, a little belligerently, who has died of AIDS? And I thought, okay, you want to know, well actually Douglas died of AIDS, and George died of AIDS, Geoffrey died of AIDS. I said Anna, Katie's mum from Positively Women, died of AIDS. I said Sheila has AIDS. She really loves Sheila and Laura and she said 'Sheila?' And I went on, yes, remember every time you went to visit Sheila in hospital? I told her Kate was HIV positive and she wanted to know if Kate would get AIDS and die. So I explained that no, she's HIV positive and if you're HIV positive you could get AIDS, and I explained as simply as I could about cells fighting things in your body and she was really attentive and interested. It was a good atmosphere to talk about it in because there were all the speeches and songs and waving of flowers. She did ask me if I were HIV positive but I pretended I hadn't heard because that was just too much. My main fear for her is first of all that she would get worried if I got a cold or flu. She's been on her own with me all her life so she's a mixture of amazing independence and dependence on me. We're very, very close and I think I'd like to keep that stress away from her as long as I can. Secondly, and just as important, she and most other children in her situation don't have access to any peer support. When my mum had cancer she could talk about it in school and with her friends, many of whom had a granny, friend, aunt or mother who also had cancer. She won't be able to do that with HIV or AIDS until the stigma's removed.

I think it's of growing importance to set up groups for children of parents who are HIV or have AIDS or have died of AIDS. It might be a tiny bit easier to tell her if there were such groups. They would have to be set up and organized in a way which was right and had a good atmosphere. Over 50 per cent of the women attending Positively Women are mothers so there's no doubt that there are an awful lot of kids around who's mums are positive. Some of those children are positive themselves.

If there is one thing all this has given me it is a love of life

- to me living every moment with happiness and optimism is paramount. I no longer take anything or anyone for granted. I have learned that I am my own best friend, I know where I stand with myself, and I trust myself completely. I have made my peace with those I love - including G - he called me two months ago and we were able to look at each other and say 'I love you' - and I do love him, my way. I will carry on working and fighting for the rights of women with HIV and AIDS and for anything I feel passionately about. I feel it is my duty and purpose in life not to be quiet, but to speak out. My responsibility for my child, whom I'll adore forever.

LEIGH

Leigh is thirty-nine, lives in Chelsea and works at Positively Women. She would love to have a country cottage with her own horse, a nice man, and lots of holidays abroad.

I WAS BORN in January 1953, the second of four children. Growing up, I did all the usual girlie stuff, ballet and tap dance, riding and so on. I wasn't terribly interested in school but I did quite well without trying too hard. My childhood was comfortable and happy, although I had a major feeling of being unloved. I don't think this was true in reality, but it was definitely how I felt at the time.

By the time I was thirteen I realized there was something very definitely going wrong with the family - my parents had separated, my mother was becoming unwell, and my father was drinking extremely heavily. I felt like my whole world had turned upside down. My mother had cancer and was literally wasting away and I never knew if my dad would be sober or drunk. He was like Jekyll and Hyde and I used to get very angry and shout and scream at him. Eventually he went into a residential alcoholic unit but was back drinking on his first day out. When I was fifteen my mother died and my father went bankrupt, which in turn led to us losing our home. One day we were living in a beautiful big house with every comfort and the next day it was gone. I went into three different childrens' homes but ended up being asked to leave each one of them. By the time I was sixteen I was living on my own.

The first drug I ever took was when I was fifteen and it was one of my father's Mandrax - I can't remember if he offered

153

or I asked - anyway that's how it started, taking Mandies and drinking whisky with my dad. I wasn't so angry with him and the world all of a sudden. I started smoking dope and taking speed at the same time, and also taking a lot of LSD.

Right from the start my drug taking was excessive. I really loved the fact that I only had to swallow smoke or snort something and it would change my mood instantly - brilliant! For a long time I enjoyed taking drugs, but that's all I ever did with my life. It never occurred to me to think about a career, further education or anything other than getting stoned, so that's all I did. It was fun for a while.

I was very talented, very creative. I would start projects, jobs, college courses, do well, show real ability, but repeat the same pattern: blow it, mess it up before it could mess up on me. I guess I didn't trust life but I did trust the drugs - they worked every time, I could rely on them.

I didn't really notice what was happening to my life. I took drugs and lived the same kind of lifestyle for twenty years, so I wasn't really aware of the decline. Gradually I started doing all the things I never thought I'd do. When I was young and first starting out on my drug career, I thought I'd never take heroin, but of course it wasn't too long before I did and when I did, I thought, 'Ah, but I'll never fix it or get a habit' and of course I did.

There were lots of times when I tried to stop, usually by substituting another drug, but I was never successful. I might manage it for a few weeks, but would always start again. Lots of friends died over the years from overdoses and my world was slowly becoming smaller. I was becoming a slave to the drugs and I was going out stealing, forging cheque books and cards, anything to get money for more drugs.

My life had become a nightmare and a long way from my original, naive, idealistic view of it being some sort of quest for enlightenment through getting high. I was now on an ever revolving merry-go-round: get up, have a hit, go out - ducking and diving and putting my liberty on the line day after day -

all to get enough money together to score. If it was a good day, I'd get some cocaine as well as smack, go home, take it, feel okay for an hour or so, and then start the whole cycle over again.

Soon, I was ending up in prison cells and spent time in Holloway on three occasions. One time my boyfriend came to visit me in prison and maybe it was because I hadn't seen him for a few weeks, but suddenly I realized he wasn't looking well. I put it down to the drugs and not looking after himself properly. But when I came home he was taken to hospital with pneumonia from which he never seemed to recover fully. The hospital ran various tests on him and he went for the results the day before Christmas Eve 1986. When he came home, I could see something was very wrong and when I asked him what it was he said he had cancer. 'Don't be ridiculous,' I said, 'it's not cancer, it's AIDS.' He said, 'Yes.' I think I'd been half joking and didn't really expect him to say yes. Although I was extremely shocked and scared, I was aware of AIDS and knew that we were in a high risk category, but of course I never really dreamt it would affect me.

It was the most horrible Christmas I've ever had: I had flu and a very painful abscess on my tooth. We had enough heroin to last us through Christmas but it wasn't taking the pain away. I knew it was highly unlikely I had escaped having the virus. I was very scared; at the that time there was a lot of publicity about AIDS and it was like, bad news! Everywhere it seemed they were saying HIV=AIDS=Death. I needed to tell someone so I chose my sister. She was scared, too scared to even come over and pick up her Christmas presents which really hurt me.

After Christmas was over I went for a test myself. During the two weeks' wait for the result, I managed to get myself arrested yet again and was put in Holloway Prison on remand. Thinking it might help me get bail, I told them I was waiting for my results. In fact I was given the result in prison. I was told I was HIV positive but not to talk about it - in case it caused mass hysteria. If anyone asked, I was to pretend I had hepatitis B. I was then put into isolation and my food was passed in through the hatch. I can't think of a worse place to hear news like that. I didn't know what to do; I was feeling sick from heroin withdrawal, I was only seven stone, and in one way it would have been some sort of release if I could have died then and there. But on the other hand there was a part of me saying, 'Hold on a minute. What about my hopes and dreams?' I'd forgotten all about the fact that once upon a time I did have some. Why hadn't I noticed my life slipping away? Is this what it had come to - being junk sick and told I had a life threatening illness while in a prison cell?! God, it felt like my whole life (or the waste of it) was hitting me all at once. What a mess I'd made of it all.

I went to court a few days later and didn't get bail. I was taken to a police cell for a few days while waiting to go back to Holloway. This cell was really dismal, the ones at Holloway were like a holiday camp in comparison. I got severe gastroenteritis, couldn't stop being sick. I was so scared and thought, 'Well, I suppose this must be it, I'm going to be constantly ill until I die, what a future!' After they transferred me back to the Holloway hospital wing, I got a bit better and then it was time to go back to court and try for bail again. There's a waiting room in Holloway where everyone sits waiting to be taken to court. However, I had to sit in a cubicle on my own for hours, listening to police officers refusing to take me to court, saying they'd heard about me, and that the last cell and van I'd been in had to be fumigated! God, I felt like a leper. Eventually I got to court and thank god, I got bail.

The next couple of years weren't easy ones because I'd become so aware of where my addiction had led me. On the one hand I wanted to do something about it, but on the other I wanted to get as stoned as possible in order to blot out the reality of my situation. What I did manage to do was get on a methadone prescription through my local drug dependency unit and that helped me to stabilize my life a bit. I put on a little weight, I stopped doing so much crime, I stayed at home more and went to my hospital appointments. For years my only contact with people was other drug users. At the hospital and at the drug dependency unit I was meeting people who weren't addicts, who lived fairly normal lives.

So my life got marginally better, but as drug taking was no longer such a twenty-four hour job, I began to realize and experience how empty my life was. There was no joy, no direction, no motivation, and most of all, no hope. My life centred on waiting for the chemist to open each morning.

One day, quite out of the blue, I'd had enough. That day I got very drunk and just realized clearly that my friends put their drugs before people and that's exactly what I had done for years too. I ended up at the drug dependency unit, asking my doctor to help me come off drugs. Afterwards I went home and collapsed in my boyfriend's arms, sobbing my heart out. It was such a relief to admit that I had a problem and needed help.

A few months later I went to a 12 Step Treatment Centre in the country for six weeks and then on to a half-way house for six and a half months.

Right. Now for the good news: I haven't had a drink or a drug for two and three quarter years. My life has changed completely. I'm definitely the healthiest I've ever been. I've cut down from smoking twenty-five cigarettes a day to one or two and am in the process of giving up altogether - I even manage without one at all on some days. I've started swimming, riding and aerobics and I feel good.

I am working full-time for Positively Women and although sometimes I find it emotionally draining, most of the time it's interesting, challenging and fulfilling. The job is varied: I facilitate support groups, do telephone and one-to-one counselling, and home and hospital visits. I work with drug users and on drug issues and go into Holloway Prison to do awareness sessions with the prisoners. I really enjoy that part of the job, as obviously I have a strong personal interest, not the least because it makes me so aware of how my life has turned around.

I think I'm pretty good working in these areas because my own personal experience gives me a deep and clear understanding of the issues.

I was taking AZT but stopped after nine months. I don't want to take it right now. Of course there's a possibility that my views might change if I get ill, but for now I don't want to swallow something which might be toxic several times a day when I don't know what it does to me, especially as I'm really quite healthy. Drugs like AZT haven't been tested long enough. We already know there are side-effects but no one is sure about what the long term ones are.

Anyway, I'm far more interested in things like acupuncture, aromatherapy, shiatsu and spiritual healing. I would much rather put my belief into alternative healing than into a chemical drug. I'm also interested in knowing more about the Bach Flower remedies which are supposed to work on an emotional level, as I know without a doubt that I've got emotional blocks which I need help with. It's important for me to work on the emotions because I know that's what fucked me up most of my life, and as far as I'm concerned my emotional well-being is connected to my physical well-being. Changing deeply engrained thinking and behavioral patterns is a pretty tall order and isn't something that can be achieved over night but I'm gradually getting somewhere with the help of my counsellor, a 12 Step programme and my higher power. In fact, today I can say that I'm beginning to love myself a little bit.

Overall, I think the important thing is being comfortable with my decisions and choices about what enhances my well being. There is less stress and strain if I'm happy about my health care choices and I know that's a good thing.

I'm conscious that the life I've led hasn't contributed to me being physically very fit but I'm working on that by starting aerobics and riding. I believe the virus contributes to feeling tired so I make sure I get enough sleep. Anyway, I can't function otherwise!

I'm not great on diet, although I'm much more aware of what

I eat these days and try to avoid total crap. Obviously eating healthily, like exercise, is good for you. Years ago I was macrobiotic and I still think that's a really good diet, but for now it's more important not be too excessive. Being completely wrapped up in something isn't balanced and could be another obsessive pattern to fall into. In any case, I haven't got the time and I enjoy eating out in good restaurants too much.

On the whole I have a very optimistic approach to living with HIV. Of course I get scared sometimes and wonder what the future holds, especially as time goes on and others around me get AIDS and become ill. But in some ways even that has helped me; it makes me have a pretty sharp focus on life, on what I want to do, on what's right or wrong for me and what's important. Certainly, the quality of my life has improved 100 per cent. Even so, sometimes I feel I need more balance in my life, as I find myself doing so much, cramming it all in, just in case!

For me there definitely is life beyond an HIV diagnosis and it's up to me to make it the best possible kind of life. On good days it is just that. On bad days it requires a lot of strength and effort. But all in all, I'm not going to sit back and be a victim. I'm going for it!

I value and love my life today. I don't think I'm scared of death although I certainly fear getting ill. There's so much I want to do and experience, and I'm not going to let having a life threatening illness get in the way of that. But it affects me. Hardly a day goes by when I don't think about it on one level or another. But maybe that's why everything seems much more precious to me these days.

SUZANNE

Suzanne was one of the original members
of Positively Women.
She died on 4 May 1989.

I'D STOPPED DRUGS the month before I got pregnant. I was
clean and off drugs for some time. I looked after my child until
just before she was three, and then I got busted for hashish. Two
weeks before my probation was finished, my parents took me
to court for custody of my daughter. From there they took my
rights as a parent away. I left and started travelling. I travelled to southeast Asia - Thailand, Malaysia, India, Pakistan,
and started taking drugs again. I was gone for four months until
I returned to England. I stopped the drugs when I arrived back;
I took the last amphetamine and then I just stopped. When I
got here I realized something was wrong with my body.

I got my diagnosis in 1985, just two months after arriving
back in England. I didn't know anything about AIDS. Once
in India, I read that in America, I don't know how many thousands had AIDS, but my English was so bad I only thought 'First
Aid', and couldn't understand what was being said in the article. I think when I got back to England, Rock Hudson had
just died. When they told me I was positive, I just thought,
'Okay, I'm dying now. That's it.' It was a shock to the system.

I was still living in a house in Brixton with some other people
and I rushed back and told them, 'AIDS, I've got AIDS!' They
were sitting there drinking tea and just looked at me without
saying anything. Then my lover came back from work and when
I told him, he was really annoyed I hadn't told him first. That
was understandable but I couldn't help it, I had to say some-

thing.

Telling the people in the house was a very stupid thing to do. I soon realized that and four weeks later I had a big party with champagne, pretending it was all a big mistake. Everybody bought it, because a year ago when I was diagnosed with full-blown AIDS, I told some of the same people and they couldn't believe it.

Now I've lost contact with a lot of those people. I write to friends every Christmas and at Easter to let them know I'm still alive. Last summer I wrote to one friend saying, 'You don't need to be afraid because I'm ill, you know', and she phoned me straight away. I think she was quite offended because she said, 'I'm coming over', but I haven't heard anything for the last month. So I think it really offended her. But I'm still going to keep on doing it, to let them know I'm still around.

When I found out, I wasn't working; then I did a job as a cleaner, and next I got a job as an auxiliary nurse. For that job I had to have a blood test. I was a little bit worried about it but I wasn't tested for HIV. It was hard because I was working in a hospital operating theatre and I heard all the jokes and could see how the medical profession actually behaves behind the backs of HIV positive patients. Obviously they didn't know I was positive and I couldn't say anything. I often thought I'd like to scream out, 'Well, fuck, you've been working with me for two years, there's nothing to be frightened of really.' Yeah, that was strange, a little bit weird.

I got ill quite suddenly. Even afterwards I thought I could fight it, get better. But I realized after some months that I wasn't going to go back to the old state of fitness. I slowly got aches and a rash and eczema - just tiredness. Now I go from one day to the other. For me AZT seemed to work quite well for nearly a year, but now the side-effects are too bad, so it seems I have to stop it. For the last two years I've also been using homeopathic treatments and herbs. The homeopathic treatment helped me a great deal with lots of small things - pain in the legs, eczema, and so on.

There's been a big difference for me between knowing I'm HIV positive and then knowing I've got AIDS. During the last year, especially in the last three or four months, I've had to adjust mentally to being more dependent on people for doing things for me. During the two years I was HIV positive, I was okay. It bothered me, but life went on and I still felt the same. I could go on as normal and work every day. Nowadays I'm thankful because I know things could be much worse, but nevertheless, during the last year I've had to adjust again and again to new disabilities. I find that very depressing.

Most of the time I think I'm all right, but when the weather is bad I nearly always get pretty depressed. Your mind is fine, it's just your body won't do what you want it to do. You can't do the simplest things like going shopping or getting on the tube. That's a big adventure!

My family all know about me - my mother, my father, and my sister. I told my mother two years ago when I found out I was HIV positive, and then when I got full-blown AIDS I told her too. She had to talk to someone, so she told my sister and that's quite difficult because they don't live in this country and they worry. It's difficult, I think, for an outsider to understand. I don't think they have anyone professional who can explain things to them. Also there's my daughter. She knows that I'm ill but it's not easy for her. She realizes that there's something more going on than just being ill. My daughter accepts me now. Last year I was over there visiting, and I was reasonably fit. I hadn't seen her for a while but, as I said, she has accepted me and now she phones sometimes. How far she will go is up to her really. I suppose it's difficult for her to think, okay, she's ill. She was really determined to stop me smoking when I was visiting.

Having the virus affected the relationship with my boyfriend. For the first two years he ignored it completely and it didn't hit him until I got really ill. But even after that, he seemed to think, 'Oh, she's going to get all right again.' It's actually in the last few months when I've been living on my own that he's realized a bit more the reality of my situation. He put a lot of pressure on me when we were living together, expecting to get his clothes washed and dinner cooked, and I just couldn't do it anymore. He has changed a lot really, but you can't change a person completely. He is definitely more easy going now. On the sexual side it's funny, because he's still approaching me and I don't know, sex is the last thing I can think of. Even if I feel desire for five or ten seconds, well, I get out of breath if I even lean down! I can't even think of wanking anymore.

When we were having sex it was safer sex, but it was always me who insisted and had to take responsibility for it. It doesn't turn you on - safe sex, or leaflets on safe sex - does it? But what does safe sex really mean? That's a question I couldn't figure out for quite a while. Okay, condoms, but if you use oil or creams... nobody told me that they could cause the bloody things to split! You have to use special water-based stuff with condoms, but I didn't know that, and I felt guilty that the condoms dissolved. Then at last, somebody told me. I'd never used condoms in my life and then the stupid things just blew away.

In the beginning I didn't want to see any counsellors but then my boyfriend and I went to see one together. The first thing she asked was, 'Are you feeling guilty?' and then she went on to say, 'You poor thing'. I didn't want pity. I didn't like her at all so I never saw her again. I couldn't tell anyone. After about two years I contacted Positively Women and that was the first time I really talked to some other people about being positive. I don't see anyone from the old times. Last week I got a letter from somebody I used to know, asking me to go for a drink, but I'm going to ignore her because there's no point in going and ending up answering stupid questions, maybe getting the 'three years' attitude. It's weird, right. One friend of my boyfriend has seen me a lot and he's suspecting something, but I'm just not admitting it. But it's getting harder to hide it, especially during the last three months. When I was HIV positive it didn't bother me so much but now I'm in a stage where

I can't hide it anymore because I look skinnier and don't walk very well. People ask questions and I don't know what to say.

It becomes more and more difficult to lie, because you're so often in hospital, always looking for new ways of treatment, looking for solutions. It's such a big part of your life that you can't hide it anymore, or pretend. You think in terms of AIDS, and eating and doing things to keep you going. Sometimes I get calls from people who don't know and I have to switch to a different planet.

In reality I do nothing. I sit in the flat staring at the TV, trying to get three square meals on a plate each day. It's so difficult to think about the future. I dream about what I would do if I were healthy or even just feeling a little bit better. Otherwise you can only really live from one day to the other. You really don't know what will be happening in four weeks' time. Maybe some bloody virus or infection will hit you. I'm spending about two days each week in hospital, just for check-ups, drugs, testing. You can't plan anything. I've tried to think of a hobby I could do that doesn't take too much energy, but I haven't found the right one yet.

I think I was the first woman diagnosed with AIDS in my borough. I was one of the first women at the hospital. Because I got practical help quite quickly and I also think it was because I was a woman. Maybe I was fortunate in having the right people around. Perhaps women react differently from men to being HIV positive or having AIDS. Maybe they need a different way of accepting it and of talking to each other. That's why I think there are more and more different groups for positive people starting up. People are not happy with only one kind of group because there are so many different ways of life.

This is true even for women. Just because you're a woman you can't expect to be absolute mates with all the rest of the women in the world. I don't know if it's a problem or not, but I can see that there are more and more groups trying to deal with different experiences - of gays, straights, women, drug users. I've been at Terrence Higgins Trust and it was quite weird to be the only woman in the room. I felt I was intruding on other people's privacy somehow. Even now that I've got to know more people who are positive, it's still very different. Just because you've got AIDS or HIV doesn't mean you should have to get on with everybody else who has got it.

It's a strange thing, this positive thinking. Sometimes it's so bloody hard to accept it. I feel strongly that AIDS is the reality. I had some old neighbours who came and visited me, two old ladies who know what's wrong with me. One of them is quite bright, but the other one said to me, 'Ah, you're giving up, look at you.' It's so fucking unbelievable - but she just didn't understand. It made me angry. How long do you go on fighting? I don't want to feel that if I get ill, it's my fault because I'm not being strong enough or thinking positively enough.

Sometimes I get quite scared. A few weeks ago when I had a really bad temperature, I was lying in bed and I got really frightened. I didn't know what to do. Fortunately I've got the Lifeline telephone, I can press the button any time and somebody will be there. But I wasn't sure what to do because I dread going into hospital and had only got out two days before. I thought, shit, you could just die. Sometimes I get to the stage where I seem to have no life force, no energy, and I think if I don't sleep I'll drift off, I'll just pop off. That's how it feels. I don't know if it would actually happen but that's the feeling and it frightens me.

At times like that I try to use breathing techniques. I try not to let the frightened feeling take over, because then maybe I'd get to a stage where I really did pop off. I try to think of every day, simple things - I'm going to stand up, eat breakfast. Then I feel all right for maybe two hours, and then everything is gone again. I'm so knackered, having just washed up some dishes and eaten breakfast and I lie down again and sleep. That's the frustrating thing.

When I think of other women who are HIV positive or have AIDS my advice is to keep holding on. That's all I can say, try to see the good things that there are. Okay, it's easy to say, but there is always someone who is much worse off than yourself. I think about the poor kids in Africa, how skinny they are through having nothing to eat. I can still drag myself outside. I can still walk on my own two feet. But walking is hard and it bothers me because everyone can see it. Otherwise I'm all right. Try to find some forms of treatment for yourself which you think are right. That's very hard, to listen to your body. There are so many different approaches, alternative ways, and technological ways, but it's finding what makes you feel better which is important. Stay in contact with the outside world, with people. It's important that you've got people you can phone. If you get too low or weak and you have to rely on people, it's important to accept that. I found it very difficult to accept people doing things for me. Most of the time I clear up before somebody comes in to clean up properly!

It's also important to sort something out about practical assistance. Things like help with the shopping, and cleaning because there are not many possibilities around. Housing is a very big factor. I was so lucky because I got a council flat, and when I got worse, I got this flat. I'm fortunate that I'm living in sheltered housing. It's all the luxury I can imagine. It's such a big relief. It takes a lot of stress away if your housing situation is all right and that's true for everyone.

HOW HIV/AIDS AFFECTS WOMEN'S LIVES

THE UK DECLARATION OF THE RIGHTS OF PEOPLE WITH HIV AND AIDS

THIS DECLARATION IS made by people with HIV and AIDS and by organizations dedicated to their welfare. The Declaration lists rights which all citizens of the United Kingdom, including people with HIV and AIDS, enjoy under international law; the Declaration then prescribes measures and recommends practices which the writers of the Declaration believe are the minimum necessary to ensure that these rights are respected and protected within the United Kingdom.

THE DECLARATION
All citizens of the United Kingdom, including people with HIV and AIDS, are accorded the following rights under international law:

* the right to liberty and security of person
* the right to privacy
* the right to freedom of movement
* the right to work
* the right to housing, food, social security, medical assistance and welfare
* the right to marry
* the right to found a family
* the right to education

These rights exist in international treaties* which the United Kingdom Government has agreed to uphold. But these rights, as they apply to United Kingdom citizens with HIV and AIDS, have not been adequately respected or protected. We therefore make a public Declaration of the Rights of People with HIV and AIDS and of our commitment to ensuring that they are upheld.

* The relevant treaties, which the UK Government has agreed to uphold, are the International Covenant of Civil and Political Rights, the International Covenant of Economic, Social and Cultural Rights (1976), the European Convention on Human Rights (1953) and the European Social Charter (1965).

For more information and/or copies of the complete Declaration please contact:
NATIONAL AIDS TRUST,
14th FLOOR, EUSTON TOWER,
286 EUSTON ROAD,
LONDON NW1 3DN.
071- 383 4246

AN AIDS CONSULTANT'S
APPROACH
TO HIV AND AIDS

DANIELLE MERCEY

Danielle Mercey is thirty-three, and works as a consultant genito-urinary physician with a special interest in women and HIV. She lives in London and has two daughters.

AS A CONSULTANT in genito-urinary medicine I see HIV positive men and women patients, and I have a particular interest in women who are HIV positive. I've been seeing women for about three years now which is as long as I've been working at this clinic. I chose to work here partly because of my interest in HIV infection. Since starting at the clinic, I have seen an increasing number of HIV positive people, although at the beginning I only saw women occasionally. Because a lot of positive women were indicating that they preferred seeing a woman doctor, my female colleagues and I had more and more women referred to us. Then, quite by chance, I made links with Positively Women and they started referring patients to this clinic.

Most clinics separate HIV positive clients from the general genito-urinary ones; talking to someone who has just found out they're HIV positive or who has an HIV related illness requires more time and therefore longer appointments. The general genito-urinary clinics are busy, in-out places, and appointments often last only ten or twenty minutes. But even when we allowed more time for our positive patients, most were still men which meant the women were being fitted in between the male patients. It sometimes meant they were sitting in the male waiting areas which for some women was not particularly suitable. Although some women didn't mind, others found it very uncomfortable. My senior registrar and I decided there was sufficient demand for a clinic specifically for positive women and that is what we set up.

Because of space constraints we cannot offer all the facilities we would like. It would be wonderful to be able to offer a crèche to the women who have children, but there is nowhere in the building to fit it in. Fortunately, there is now a clinic at Great Ormond Street hospital which accommodates children and is run in conjunction with a paediatrician. There, children and babies can be seen at the same appointment as their mother.

The general principles of care for someone who is HIV positive start before a person has an HIV test with good pre-test counselling. Why does someone want to have a test? How is it going to alter them to know they are positive? Who are they going to tell if they are positive? How might it affect their work or their relationships? Will it have implications for their children?

These principles then extend to the giving of the results, and, if we assume a positive result, the after-care that follows from it. Giving the result and offering back up and support in the immediate phase after someone discovers they're positive are important, vital aspects of care. They will remain the same no matter what changes in relation to possible future treatments. Follow up interviews to answer questions that patients invariably come up with in the few weeks after they discover they're positive are important too. What does it mean for them and for the future? What are their chances of life? What can we as doctors tell them about the likelihood of developing an illness? What is the likelihood of their dying? All of these questions and the discussions arising from them form basic principles of care.

The management of someone who is essentially well and HIV positive comes next. Although they don't have any specific HIV-associated illness, they may have minor problems from time to time. For instance they may notice changes in the condition of their skin, or they may be more susceptible to feeling tired. Our role at this point is to give advice about maintaining general health in terms of nutrition, exercise, sleep, and to treat each condition as it arises. Doctors in the clinic also monitor the patients for signs of immune suppression.

Increasingly people are talking about intervention at an earlier stage; opinions really differ over the question of early medical intervention and not surprisingly, practice differs also. It is now universally accepted that one of the ways of monitoring patients is through the T-cell count. The T-cell count becomes the magic touchstone and if it falls below a certain number, then many in the medical profession believe you should be treated with an anti-viral such as zidovudine (AZT). Patients also should have appropriate treatment to prevent pneumocystis carinii pneumonia (PCP) which can greatly reduce its danger to HIV positive patients.

In this country, zidovudine is now licensed for use in patients who have very low T-cell counts. However, that does not automatically mean doctors are saying that if you are well but your T-cell count is below a certain number, you should be on zidovudine. There are still differences of opinion and practice between hospitals. At one London clinic zidovudine might be prescribed for low T-cell counts, and not at another. I would like to think that the known relative benefits and risks of anti-viral therapy were discussed with every patient, and that they then could make their own decision about what to do. This would be the ideal practice. However, if I'm honest, I have to say that the way a doctor discusses any treatment with a patient influences that patient's ultimate decision. It's very difficult to say, 'Right, go away and read these papers and come back and tell me what you think you want to do', because the most commonly asked question is, 'Well, what do you think, doctor?' You have to give your opinion. You don't have to maintain that it's automatically the right opinion, but based on the evidence you know about, you have to state what you think. Inevitably this leads to difference in practices between hospitals. One of the most controversial areas in HIV/AIDS medicine is how and when doctors intervene when HIV positive people are essentially well.

The large Concorde trial, which is still underway, may be able to give us better information on which to base these decisions. At the moment, the two major types of intervention are zidovudine, the anti-viral treatment, and the so-called primary prophylaxes which are used to stop specific infections before they occur. One of the most commonly used is a prophylaxis against PCP. My feeling is that this sort of primary intervention is something we should be offering people at an early stage; the risk of taking the prophylaxis is minimal and the benefit is definite: you can delay the onset of the pneumonia which otherwise can be dangerous in a person who is HIV positive.

Then there is the management of the patient who doesn't have AIDS but who is ill in some way related to their HIV status. Then the management is of the condition: for instance, if it's diarrhoea, it's management of diarrhoea. Investigations to look for underlying causes would start and treatment would follow, either of the cause or, if no cause were found, symptomatic treatment. As well, there might be treatment with anti-viral therapy. For some of the non-specific features associated with HIV infection, treatment with an anti-viral therapy which acts against the HIV, can sometimes help the symptoms. For instance, patients who have lost a lot of weight may regain it if they start on zidovudine.

Then there is the management of a patient who has an AIDS-defining condition. Quite often that illness initially has to be treated in hospital. If a patient gets PCP or cryptococcal meningitis, the chances are they will be admitted to hospital, both for an investigation of the condition and initially at least, for the treatment. At our clinic when a patient is admitted to hospital they are looked after by a different set of doctors while they are there. But we maintain very close contact. We visit the patients and we're all present when the patients' cases are discussed on a weekly basis. It isn't as discontinuous as it may sound and it isn't the same in all hospitals, but often there are different doctors looking after a person as an out-patient and as in-patient.

Once the patient has recovered from an initial acute infection or whatever the problem is, they would continue to be seen by us as an out-patient at the clinic. The difference then is that we would be probably see the patient more frequently in order to monitor their therapies more closely. Also, because some-one who has had one AIDS-defining diagnosis may have a higher chance of going on and developing another complication of HIV, we would want to keep a closer check on them.

My relationship with each individual patient's own GP is variable. Some patients haven't got a GP and don't want one; therefore a doctor at the clinic acts as their GP. However, we encourage patients to find one because GPs have a very important role in any patient's care, particularly for someone who may develop a long-term illness. Some patients feel they can't tell their GP they are positive because the doctor is a family friend and the patient is concerned about confidentiality. In that case we usually suggest helping them change their GP. We have contacted general practice surgeries on behalf of patients and said, 'We have a patient who is HIV positive, would you be prepared to take them on your list?' The response gives us a good idea of the practice's attitude. If the answer is 'Of course, someone who is HIV positive needs a GP as much as anyone else. We have spaces', then that's fine. If it's an immediate, 'Oh well, we haven't got very many spaces, we think we're a bit full...', then we tend not to bother. We don't want to put our patients in an unpleasant or awkward position. Now we know who the interested GPs are, so we know better who to ask. I think that GPs are increasingly taking an interest; they do want to know how to help the patients.

The HIV positive people we see at this clinic are a diverse group. However, because of our central London location we do look after a group of predominantly middle-class, highly educated, professional, white gay men, who read the medical literature. They don't just read the *Pink Paper*, they come along with their copy of the *Lancet* and say 'What do you think about this trial? I was a bit concerned that the confidence interval seems very wide on this result, do you think it's reliable?' It's kept us doctors on our toes, which is no bad thing. It can be very stimulating for a doctor to have discussions with well-informed patients about the ethics of doing a placebo-controlled trial. But not all patients can have, or want to have, that sort of understanding. Risk and probability are quite sophisticated concepts and not everybody understands them; people may not grasp the ideas of the chance of success of one treatment compared to another. To a certain extent, I think you have to modify what you do say and base it on what you think the understanding of your patient is. But having said that, I'm sure that in the past doctors have underestimated what patients can understand.

It's been amazing to me the extent to which patients can make informed decisions about their treatment. Of course you have to be satisfied that their decision is based on correct information and that in simplifying information you have not biased it one way or another. For instance, if you say that a drug has a 98 per cent chance of giving side-effects, it might mean that most patients will feel tired the first afternoon they take the pill and after that are fine, or, it might mean that 98 per cent of the patients on that medication will need a blood transfusion. These are two very different situations. It's very easy for the person delivering information to influence the recipients perception of it. Increasingly, this is an area where the press and other information-giving bodies who are not directly medical have helped. Maybe what they've put out hasn't always been 100 per cent accurate, but they have tried to understand what we are doing and why we are doing it, and to put it across to people in a way that allows them to make informed choices.

If there is one good thing that has come out of the HIV epidemic, it's been the way a lot of medical attitudes have been challenged. For example, take the whole business of HIV testing. I've heard so many doctors say, 'But we don't get a person's informed consent to do a chest x-ray, and that might show they've got lung cancer.' Well, maybe we should get informed consent from a patient before we do a chest x-ray. Perhaps HIV testing isn't so different and it's much more that all the rest of our practice has been wrong up until now.

Access to drugs and treatments which haven't been tested thoroughly has been a terribly difficult area for doctors and people with HIV infections. One of the anti-viral drugs being tested and used is didanosine (Dideoxy inosine or DDi). The North American trials include a few hundred patients, whereas their expanded access programme, which allows anyone who is eligible to receive DDi, has several thousands of people taking it. That does have unfortunate consequences. It means that the information we should be able to gain from all the people taking DDi is not being collected. So for people in the future there will be unanswered questions about the use of DDi. For example: What is the rate at which side effects occur? How effective is it at preventing progression to AIDS or at prolonging life? The major HIV drug trials which are happening in this country are coordinated by the Medical Research Council (MRC). There are now two major drug trials being conducted - the Concorde trial which is looking at the use of AZT in a symptomatic patients, and the Alpha trial which is looking at the use of didanosine. A further combination anti-viral trial is to start soon.

Both the Concorde and the Alpha trials now have a lay representative on their working party from one of the patient groups. That person will have been involved in the very early designs of the trial. For example, from a strictly scientific view, in the didanosine trial it is ethical to compare using didanosine against using nothing, because you cannot say that either group is disadvantaged. (At this point we don't know if di-danosine is going to work - we've got the theoretical evidence about why it should, but nobody can say that didanosine is an effective drug to use in someone who is HIV positive.) However, this was not what the patients' groups wanted. They wanted the right to take didanosine if they wanted to. The Alpha trial bowed to that pressure, and divided the trial into two parts. One could opt either to go into the part where one had a one-in-three chance of taking dummy pills, or go into the other arm of the trial which guarantees that the participant receives didanosine and compares high and low doses. This appears to have won approval from the patient groups; they feel that we've been sensitive to their demands. The downside is that most patients are going to opt for the no-placebo (dummy) arm, and that means that we are not actually doing a trial to say whether didanosine works or not, because we can only compare whether a high dose or a low dose is better. It may be that neither low nor high dosages are any better than taking nothing, but that will be very hard to prove. This may delay the use of other drugs, or it may mean that we'll use the drug inappropriately for a while; as I said, it is a very difficult area.

Another difficult area concerns effective dosage levels of zidovudine. There is no evidence from trials that lower doses are as effective. There is some evidence comparing lower doses with very high does (higher than we use, anyway) that indi-cates that at very high doses people experience intolerable side-effects. We have known that for quite a while and it is the reason why we don't use the very high doses any more. There isn't a specific trial in this country comparing doses. The prob-lem is that if you have a limited number of patients, you can't run a hundred different trials on everything; you don't have enough people and you need to have quite large numbers of patients to see differences. The more treatments are refined, the smaller the differences in outcome you expect to see are. It's not as if one drug is going to be 100 per cent effective and everyone on it will feel fine, live forever, and without it get sick and die within two years. That sort of comparison isn't happening any more. It's more about whether a drug makes people live an extra six months; does it make them feel a little bit better at that time? These are all very subtle differences. Statistically, to prove those differences you need large numbers of people. At the moment we don't feel that there is enough justification for giving low does of zidovudine. In other words, there is not enough evidence that they are effective. If someone can tolerate what we would call 'full dose', which is one gram a day, then we see no reason for altering their treatment. It's different when someone can't tolerate a full dose, because then we would be perfectly happy to try them on a lower one if that meant they could take at least some zidovudine.

A lot of patients want to try alternative medicines, and it would be totally wrong of me to arrogantly say that they shouldn't or couldn't. I would not discourage patients from trying alternative remedies while there is no complete answer to the problems of HIV infection. I always ask patients to discuss alternative treatments with me because I'm concerned that occasionally people have been subject to fraudulent claims about treatments. For instance, some HIV positive patients have been advised to try diets which are deficient in nutrients, which is dangerous. If there were anything that I thought was potentially hazardous, then I would have to advise them of that. At the end of day, it's still their decision. After all they can turn around and tell me that zidovudine is potentially hazardous.

I can usually tell patients where they might seek out advice on alternative treatments and there are now sufficient people around who, within their own alternative specialty, see people who are HIV positive. A lot of the gay organizations have been very good about setting up those links. Places like the London Lighthouse have practitioners coming in to do aromatherapy, massage, and acupuncture who deal specifically with HIV patients. Why do people go to alternative practitioners whose treatments many doctors feel have never been proved, or who may offer what seems to us bizarre kinds of treatment? Why would someone prefer to go to them instead of coming and seeing me? We have to think about those questions, and I believe we have learned a lot about listening to patients, about making time to talk to them, and to hear about all of their anxieties. Rather than saying to someone, 'You've got this infection, here are the pills, see you in four months time', which was all too common in the past, doctors are beginning to look at the whole person.

We don't understand why some patients' disease progresses so much more quickly than others. We need to know more about the importance of co-factors and HIV infection. We know that there are known differences between types of HIV virus: there seems to be a more aggressive virus and a less aggressive one. But whether one changes into the other, and if so, why, isn't fully understood. The role of other infections, such as cytomegolavirus is one which has been looked at on several occasions. Do other factors such as immune suppression from other chronic infections affect things? Does the fact that you have malaria make a difference? Does malnutrition make a difference? You can show that people who are severely malnourished have some of the features of immune suppression. Do lesser degrees of malnutrition act as co-factors? I think the answer at the moment is that we just don't know.

I see a real mixture of women who are HIV positive. Some have been drug users in the past; some of them are still using drugs; some are partners of men they did not know were positive. Others are partners of men who are HIV positive drug users, HIV positive bisexuals, Africans, or haemophiliac men. There is also a group of women who were infected through unscreened blood transfusions when HIV infection was in the general population, but before it had been discovered. We are seeing increasing numbers of positive women but we often don't know when they were infected. It's worrying that we have very little feel for what's going on. We have no idea how many new people are being infected each day. There are the anonymous sero-prevalence studies underway at the moment, whereby leftover bits of blood from syphilis serology can be tested anonymously so there is no connection to the patient from whom the blood was taken. The results of these studies give us a numerical value. We can say, 'One in a hundred women who come to this clinic are HIV positive.' These anonymous tests are done at ante-natal clinics for similar reasons. We want to know what is happening in regard to HIV infection. Are people still being infected? Is anyone taking any notice of the government HIV/AIDS campaigns? If they are taking notice now, will they still take notice in five years time if nothing dramatic seems to have happened to heterosexuals by then? That is one of the big fears at the moment: you can frighten people for only so long with the picture of a heterosexual epidemic, but if it doesn't happen, what do you say?

As far as lesbians are concerned, I know from the medical literature that there were a couple of cases reported where it seemed that a woman had acquired HIV through sexual contact with another woman, and if you look at it theoretically, is possible. It could happen if you had open sores and then transmitted cervical, vaginal secretions, or blood, to someone else's open sores. The medical profession should understand that although it is unlikely for lesbians to transmit HIV to one another through woman-to-woman sexual practices, it doesn't mean that lesbians cannot be HIV positive. A number of lesbians have had heterosexual partners at some stage, or may intermittently continue to have sex with men; lesbians may have injected drugs or might have had a blood transfusion in the past.

One should not be too dogmatic when discussing risks of transmission. We're frequently asked if HIV can be transmitted through oral sex. We would love to be able to have a yes/no answer to that question, but how can we? How can we find a whole group of people who have only ever had oral sex and never had any other form of sexual contact, find out how many of those have acquired HIV, and then eliminate anyone who may have acquired it through sharing needles or anything else? It would be almost impossible to do that sort of work. We can only look at the theoretical reasons why and how HIV is transmitted, and then suggest that does or doesn't happen between women. We tend to give very practical advice about covering cuts or sores on hands, if hands are going to touch genitals, and suggest avoiding contact if someone has any open wounds.

We have questions about menstruation and HIV transmission too. If you are coming into contact with a menstruating woman's blood is the risk increased? Looking at heterosexual transmission of HIV, there seems to be contradictory evidence. Some researchers have shown that a man stands a greater chance of acquiring HIV from a woman if he has intercourse with her when she's menstruating. But another study showed no association at all. Again, theoretically, if you don't have cuts on your hands, or sores in your mouth, then even if you are coming into contact with HIV positive menstrual waste (it isn't all blood, it's blood mixed up with all sorts of other things) the actual chance of it infecting you is minimal. But nobody feels confident enough to say there is no risk, because of the potential consequences of that advice being proved incorrect. It's the same with advice about sharing sex toys. It's best to have your own and not share them, but if you do share, it's important to wash, clean, and dry the toys between sharing. It's also possible to use condoms on sex toys like vibrators or dildoes, and change the condom before sharing.

In this country safer sex is especially difficult for young people to take on. What skills does an average sixteen-year-old have to negotiate having non-penetrative sex? There was an article in the *New Statesman* reporting on young people and safer sex. To them, sex was actually 'screwing', and other things are not the 'real thing'. They even had the idea that other sexual activities were a bit weird and kinky, and they certainly would be embarrassed to ask a partner to consider doing such things. 'Straight screwing', well, that's normal, that's what people do. There is evidence that intercourse is often the least satisfying sexual activity for women, so it's ironic that in relation to safer sex, it's still seen as the only 'real' sex. There are so many ironies and contradictions. We're giving sexual advice which feminists would have been thrilled about twenty years ago, advice which emphasises a wide range of pleasurable sexual activities besides actual intercourse. There is a lot of work to be done in order to enable a whole variety of people, men, women, young people, homosexual and heterosexual, to successfully take on board the practice of safer sex.

RESEARCH: HIV AIDS AND THE INVISIBILITY OF WOMEN

EMILY SCHARF

Emily has worked over the years (both paid and voluntary) in providing support services to a range of people. She has been involved in education and training, and manages to balance, fairly happily, her split lives as City-Emily and Country-Emily.

MARCH 1992

HIV CAME INTO my life during the era of sensationalized HIV media reporting and I got involved as a volunteer, partly out of concern for myself because it was frightening and I couldn't understand what was really happening, even though I wanted to know, and partly because there was something clearly wrong in the reporting. I was hearing all the old prejudices surging up in the attempt to blame someone, or some place for the virus.

I now do freelance training for groups of people about HIV information and issues. I also continue my voluntary work which has shifted focus more and more from general issues of HIV health education and support needs, to the impact of HIV on women.

Only a few days ago I left a meeting with a Department of Health organization feeling extremely worried and angry, because yet more issues are looming in the future which will have a negative effect on women. I started writing this article at the same time.

A decade has passed since AIDS illnesses were first recognized, and yet women remain invisible. This invisibility continues despite the reality that in most parts of the world, equal numbers of women and men are affected by HIV, and despite recent publicity in Western countries about increasing numbers of women being diagnosed with AIDS.

Why are women invisible? When we begin to ask this question, we see through the 'spotlight' of HIV all the problems that exist in our societies world-wide, including the familiar ones for women. HIV highlights all the issues around women's positions in society: often poorer; less access to health care for themselves; little support in their roles as carers for others; and in less powerful positions to negotiate relationships, including the sexual aspects of relationships, most specifically safer sex.

We also see that to a great extent society's images of women have directed and limited medical and scientific HIV research, which in turn has shaped and limited the definitions of 'AIDS' and 'HIV-related conditions'. All of this contributes to women's invisibility in relation to HIV and AIDS.

Where women are visible at all, their images have often reflected society's notions of what women are: the same as men (a rib out of Adam's body!); 'mothers'; carers or partners of others; 'good women' versus 'bad women' (meaning sexually active women); innocent versus undeserving; and unable to make decisions for themselves because some one else has that power, or because they are not capable. For poor and black women, these perceived 'truths' often combine with stereotyped images of poverty and racial prejudice. Research into HIV consequences, and into HIV transmission and treatment unfortunately has reflected all of these images.

Research into the consequences and treatment of HIV has been based on research carried out largely on men. This procedure is not uncommon in medical and scientific research, but it ignores the obvious fact that women's bodies are different from men's, with a complex reproductive system, hormonal differences, body weight to fat difference, and much more. These differences affect both the consequences of having HIV and the impact of treatment drugs on women's bodies.

Much drug treatment research has excluded women because of the possible 'danger' to their reproductive role, and because they are regarded by many in the scientific community as 'non-compliant' (not to be counted on). The result of this 'unreliability' has meant in practice that often women are excluded from drug trials because social circumstances, such as the need for child care or lack of money, mean they cannot attend a clinic or hospital regularly.

Research into the transmission of HIV (how HIV passes from person to person) has included a study done in Kenya by a group of scientists from the USA, Canada, and Kenya to look at the effects of a spermicide on the transmission rate of HIV. [1] Sex workers (prostitutes) were regularly given either the spermicide application or a placebo (empty) application, and then the researchers counted the number of women in each group who became infected with HIV. (They concluded that the spermicide had caused more women to have become infected than normal.) No HIV prevention information or health education was given to the women, in order to achieve 'unbiased' results. Such research practice shows a disturbing disregard for women's lives.

However, most of the existing HIV research involving women has been based on concern about transmission to and consequences in new-born babies. Women are studied primarily in their role of mothers-to-be, and the focus of the research is clearly meant to find out the consequences to children of having an HIV positive mother. Women with HIV are often described medically as 'vectors of vertical transmission'. And we hear some professionals in the medical and scientific communities speak of the 'management' of transmission of HIV to children, i.e. the management of the mother. This management has some-times included medical professionals putting strong pressure on women with HIV to terminate their pregnancies. Both abroad and in Britain, there is an increasing call for universal HIV test-ing of all pregnant women. This seems to be in direct opposi-tion to the Department of Health's ethical stand that people have the right to make the choice about whether to be tested for HIV or not, and when. The concern we hear being expressed tends not to be for the pregnant woman, who at a time of great change might have to face the extra challenges around HIV status. It seems much more to be aimed at the medical 'management' of the child's HIV status, not through treatment necessarily, but mainly through observation and testing.

What we see by looking at HIV research is a common pat-tern in much medical research: the low priority given to women and their health needs.

How does the research which exists, with all its limits and biases, influence they understanding and defining of AIDS? AIDS (Acquired Immune Deficiency Syndrome) is actually a complicated and cumbersome medical definition or label, strongly influenced by the US Centres for Disease Control. The definition of AIDS has been expanded twice since its creation. When we look at what this AIDS definition means, this is under-standable. Presently it is a list (syndrome = collection or list) of thirty-nine 'life threatening' illnesses and conditions specific to HIV infection. Either one or a combination of these illnesses plus HIV presence is necessary in order to receive a diagnosis of AIDS. A further complication is that, although these con-ditions are supposed to be 'life threatening', some are easily treatable, some now have preventative treatment, some aren't life threatening, and some were common in certain communi-ties previous to HIV. But what makes these illnesses 'HIV specific' is that they can become severe and life threatening when HIV has damaged the immune system. Also they can affect less usual sites in the body, or persist longer than usual. This collection of thirty-nine illnesses has been based on two types of research: anecdotal published reports, based on the observations of clinicians in the HIV field; and one study in the United States of the 'natural history' of HIV, that is, the consequences of HIV in gay men who were mainly white and middle-class.[2] In other words, the present definition of AIDS is based on illnesses and conditions found in men.

WOMAN-SPECIFIC HIV RESEARCH

In general, reports and research directed at how HIV affects women are very recent, despite the fact that it has been known that women are affected in large numbers throughout the world for about eight years. Sadly, there are now large numbers of women with HIV in the United States. Published research from US medical clinicians on patterns of HIV in women are now being reported. The results are alarming:

* A USA government study showed that 48 per cent of women known to be HIV positive died of conditions not included in the AIDS definition [3]
* Women appear to live a much shorter time after diagnosis than men do
* Poor women and black women are disproportionately affected
* There appear to be patterns of illnesses and conditions resulting from the damage HIV does to the body's immune system that are specific to women's reproductive systems, and others that appear more often in women than in men. The gynaecological conditions include vaginal thrush (Vaginal Candidiasis), Pelvic Inflammatory Disease (PID), and cervical cancer, all considered 'common women's complaints', but clearly aggravated by HIV, resistant to the normal treatments and also particularly active.

Unfortunately, most of this research has not included socio-economic factors. There is a problematic division in much of the scientific community between 'pure' science, which produces 'hard facts', and social science. This divides medical research and epidemiological research (i.e. research on the movement of HIV through the populations throughout the world), from studies of social and economic factors. This division has an enormous impact on HIV research in general, and on women specifically.

Because there has not been a consideration of socio-economic factors, the published results about research on women's specific illnesses have been held up to question or debate or even discounted. They are, indeed, problematic:

* The research results are difficult to interpret. It is not clear whether these are the results of HIV infection or of socioeconomic factors such as poor housing, little money, lack of access to health care, or due to the pressures within 'traditional women's roles'. For example, women may put the care of their children or partners who may be ill, before caring for themselves. This may mean that they don't seek medical help until they are very ill.
* The research results are difficult to apply. Because it isn't clear whether the problems are medical or socio-economic, or a combination of both, it is difficult to plan and fund the needed services. Are better or more accessible medical services needed? Are new ones needed? Are more, or more flexible, support systems called for?
* The research results are difficult to transfer. For example, are the illnesses and conditions that some women experience in the USA the same for women in Britain? What part does the lack of a national health care system play in the USA research results? Are illnesses worse for women in the USA because health care is limited for people who are poor or those who don't have a job, or who are HIV positive and can't get private health insurance?

Obviously, a general study of the 'natural history' (the consequences) of HIV in women is needed. Funding for this, however, has only recently been granted in Britain and in the USA.

The studies are in the planning stages and the results will not be known for several years. Unfortunately, the British study has not included a consideration of socio-economic factors because of the added expense of including this and the attitude that an epidemiological study should gather only 'hard' facts.

Anecdotal published research from clinicians about woman-specific HIV conditions has been discounted so far by the government organizations which gather statistics and define AIDS - the Centres for Disease Control (CDC) in the USA, and the Communicable Disease Surveillance Centre (CDSC) in Britain (excluding Scotland). The information about women's conditions has been rejected even though such types of information about men, with the same limitations, were accepted. The AIDS definition remains unchanged and women remain invisible.

Throughout the world women have felt the impact of HIV on their lives. The 'absence' of women until recently in HIV research, and the invisibility of women in the current definition of AIDS, have both added a series of cascading problems:

* Women remain 'statistically insignificant', and are therefore discounted: at present the epidemiology of HIV, that is the movement of HIV through the human population of the world, is interpreted through the number of people with a diagnosis of AIDS. It is on this information that governments and departments of health base their planning and budgeting for services and support. When so many women die without receiving an AIDS diagnosis, there is a clear problem of under-reporting of the impact of HIV on women. In Britain since the number of women diagnosed with AIDS is small, women remain 'statistically insignificant'. Therefore trends concerning women cannot be determined and women are discounted.

These statistics are further biased against women by methods of gathering and sorting of the information received by the CDC and CDSC. At present, when there is more than one possible way that a woman might have contracted HIV, a method described as a 'hierarchy of transmission risks' is used to determine where a woman will be placed in the 'Mode of Transmission' statistics. This hierarchy is based on the questionable notion of 'high risk groups' rather than the understanding that it is not who we are, but what we do, that puts us at risk of HIV transmission. Heterosexual transmission is at the bottom of the hierarchy. Therefore, only if all other risks are totally non-existent will a person be placed in that category. The result is that the statistics for hetero-sexual transmission are always under-represented. And information on woman-to-woman transmission isn't even solicited.

* Women in Britain and throughout the world are diagnosed late or misdiagnosed. The AIDS definition and the classification of HIV-related symptoms and illnesses inform medical professionals throughout the world of the 'accepted' consequences of HIV. Because there are no women-specific conditions included, it is not clear to many medical practi-tioners what they should be looking for in order to ensure earlier recognition of HIV-related illnesses in women.

* Due to misdiagnosis or late diagnosis, women are excluded from important treatment and services that could enable them to have healthier and longer lives.

* The impact and side effects of drug treatments on women are untested and therefore unknown.

* The true picture of HIV within each country is distorted. This affects how prevention information is offered; where HIV research will be directed; and what the current and future health and service needs of women and women with children affected by HIV are.

* Women don't receive the information and support that allows them to take responsibility for their own lives and health, as well as for the people they may be caring for.

HOW CAN THIS BE CHANGED?
Although there are notable exceptions, governments and service

providers generally did not respond particularly rapidly or gracefully to the needs that have arisen out of HIV. A major campaign by gay men was required, one which entailed much hard work, in order to get some, often limited, level of governmental recognition of the health and service needs of gay men affected by HIV.

It is increasingly clear, however, that this limited recognition of needs has not been transferred to women affected by HIV. We need to raise a similar campaign to ensure that women become visible with the HIV picture and that services and support needed by women are provided. We need to work together to press for recognition and change in the following six areas:

1) The current AIDS Case Definition needs to be changed to include illnesses specific to women. The current classification of HIV-related illnesses also needs to include conditions specific to women, including vaginal thrush.

2) Health needs and service and support needs for women need to be clearly defined and funding provided to offer them. Issues for women as carers and for women in black and ethnic communities need especially to be addressed.

3) The recently funded British research study of HIV in women needs to include a study of socio-economic factors, in order to make the results meaningful and applicable.

4) Tests on drugs and drug treatment programmes need to include gender comparisons, and need to involve women both in the planning and in the studies themselves. Provision needs to be made in order to make drug trials accessible to women, including women caring for others.

5) A woman's right to make decisions for herself, both about HIV testing and about reproductive rights, needs to be safeguarded. Any possible violations of these, such as HIV testing without the woman's informed consent or 'universal named HIV testing of all pregnant women in high prevalence areas', need to be challenged and stopped.

6) Finally and very importantly, women who are positive and women who represent other positive women need to be

actively involved on the working committees to plan and set up any HIV research that involves women. This is particularly important in creating protocols (procedures for putting the studies into practice) and in soliciting information from women (through questionnaires, interviews, etc).

These concerns are presently being raised by women involved in the HIV and AIDS field, including the Women's HIV/AIDS Network (WHAN), London - a network of women concerned about how HIV affects women. These issues, however, need to be recognized as familiar patterns within the broader context of women's health issues. Support and co-operation from women's health organizations and women concerned about women's health, would build a broader base of awareness that HIV issues for women are part of a bigger picture. Together we can work to end the invisibility of women affected by HIV.

REFERENCES
1. Paper presented at the Fifth International AIDS Conference, Montreal, 1989. Joan Kriess from the University of Washington, Seattle, USA was the presenter. Paper reference: MAO 36.
2. The MAC Study (Multicenter AIDS Cohort Study), National Institutes for Allergy and Infectious Disease, 1985 - ongoing.
3. Chu, S. et al. 'Impact of the Human Immunodeficiency Virus Epidemic on Mortality in Women of Reproductive Age, United States', *Journal of the American Medical Association*, 11 July, 1990, 254 (4): 225-229.

A NATUROPATH'S APPROACH TO HIV AND AIDS

CAROL SMITH

Carol Smith practices naturopathy and osteopathy in London. She has been politically active in the women's movement and in health politics for many years.

I'VE CHANGED MY mind about HIV and AIDS over the past five years in relation to treatment and as a general issue. Reading the reports from the 1991 International Conference on AIDS in Italy made me start thinking all over again. It sounds dramatic but perhaps on some level a version of the world as we know it is coming to an end. How much more destruction do we need to do to the world, how much more ecological damage, how much more legally prescribed drug abuse can we perpetuate, and not see the damage? Something terrible is going on. Perhaps we need to look more openly at the question of HIV and AIDS and consider it from an entirely different perspective, in order to arrive at more successful ways of appraising and treating it. Let's look at different reasons why it is happening. I'm not really interested in what the flavour of the month is about AIDS, although of course I'm concerned and I care very much about treatment issues. But we need more than treatment in order to understand what's happening.

I don't think that people with or without HIV, immune

compromised or otherwise, should necessarily do any more to keep themselves healthy than I thought they should do fifteen years ago when I first got into health work. Basically everybody in this world has a right to physical health, good nutrition, clean water, decent housing, love, care, and affection. Everyone should have access to their spirituality and creativity. But most people don't have all these things, and that lack ultimately is going to have a seriously detrimental effect on their health. Over the past ten years, in my work as a naturopathic practitioner, I have seen, more or less, the same range of people (mainly women). Many of them are living stressed lives and are in a more dire state psychologically, emotionally, and spiritually, than they were ten years ago. Some of that manifests itself physically. I do a lot of gynaecology, and there are some 'gynaecological diseases' which I hardly ever see any more. For example, I used to see an enormous number of women with endometriosis and now I only see the odd case. Partly it's to do with what the medical profession recognizes and takes on, in other words, who gets diagnosed. Five or six years ago I had a good success rate with fibroids, and I could give a positive long-term prognosis to most women I saw. Now I have to say to women with fibroids that although I used to have a good success rate, I most certainly don't now. I think it's partly to do with global and ecological reasons, things like the interaction of different pesticides and how that relates to effects on the body's hormones. These are physical examples which relate to women, but everybody's in more of a state emotionally and spiritually; some diseases seem to occur much less, and while it's obviously better to have fibroids than HIV, nevertheless, what's changed? I haven't changed, what I do doesn't change, and I don't believe that's the problem. I see many, many, more women with ovarian cysts and many more with non-specific pelvic pain. What is non-specific pelvic pain about? The gynaecological examples are the most striking, but I also see lots of other things, such as allergies. And whatever myalgic encephalitis (ME) actually is, there are many more people with symptoms of post-viral syndrome than there were five years ago.

It's the emotional, spiritual, psychological state of the world which I find shocking. I see women in despair, they don't know where they're going, they fell off their path years ago; young women in their early twenties with their whole lives to look forward to. When I was in my early twenties, we weren't like that, and that was only eighteen years ago. Ten years of Thatcher accounts for some of it, but it doesn't fully explain the desolation of being which I see in many younger women. Why are people losing their way - a way which might be signposted with some hope or direction? Is it the lack of anything substantial to believe in? When I was a young lesbian, into radical politics, we had ideals we believed we were working for, and if I didn't still retain my revolutionary politics I might be in the same spiritual crisis I've described. This state of despair ties in to a general understanding of why things like HIV are happening now. But when I think of the practical, day-to-day treatment of HIV and AIDS, it seems to matter very little what people who have the HIV virus do in relation to keeping their health together if they are generally healthy and in a positive state of mind. The gay men I see with HIV, I see primarily for other problems like back pain or eczema. I haven't been treating them specifically for HIV and they don't want me to. They carry on with their lives and they're adamant that they're not going to get into the so-called HIV lifestyle.

In some ways, what I'm going to say now contradicts everything I believe in about alternative medicine and approaches to health. Probably it all revolves around balance and individual needs. I used to worry about the HIV positive men I see, and think 'Oh god, I wish they weren't drinking so much coffee and alcohol', but it doesn't seem to make any difference to their health status. They're happy, they're in their lives and it doesn't seem to make any difference to anything to do with HIV. You can see other people with HIV who run around popping vitamins, and there they go, slowly downhill. That's a generalization and I'm sure it's not true of everybody by any means, but it has made me think. Does it mean that if you feel emotionally good about yourself and what you're doing with your life that the rest of it, all the coffee and alcohol and smoking doesn't seem to do much harm?

People who are beginning to manifest symptoms of one of the opportunistic illnesses associated with HIV have much more reason to strengthen their immune systems. If you keep your immune system together, the odd little symptom is not going to develop as quickly as it might otherwise. For example, if people with glandular fever (another immune compromising illness) abuse themselves, they feel terrible and they don't get better. Or, if somebody who was HIV positive came to me with faint touches of oral thrush and no other symptoms I would be much keener on getting them to drop the 'bad' habits which might be impeding their recovery. But the people who come to me and are HIV positive and have no symptoms let me know within about three seconds that they're not interested in treatment to do with HIV and I respect that.

Respecting their wishes doesn't mean I have given up what I believe are sensible guidelines - in general it's sensible for people to eat fairly well, not to have billions of coffees, not to drink alcohol every night and not to smoke fifty-five cigarettes a day. If someone feels okay, on average, and has good energy, then a bit of immune abuse is no big deal - and maybe it keeps their head together and makes them happy. If it makes someone happy to sit in a cafe and drink two cups of coffee three times a week - great. But if their glands pop up all the time then it's not such a good idea. People need to have a more sensible holistic approach to how they live their lives. Everybody's more obsessed with the state of the world and more obsessed with the state of their own health, but I don't think that's necessarily a good thing. The people who need to worry tend not to, or at least push it out of their minds, and the people who don't need to worry, do.

I can hardly talk about all this without extending the discussion globally. Unless we look at the situation globally, we might as well get off the bus now. Here we are after twenty to twenty-five years of political work and what are we doing? Looking at how many cups of coffee we drink in western Europe? I mean, really, forget it.

It's a tragedy that it's primarily gay men and intravenous drug users who were affected by HIV first and in such great numbers in the West. We struggled for years and years in gay liberation and what do we get for it? Great - we get AIDS! I'm not interested in heterosexual do-good HIV workers telling gay men to use safe sex. Of course I think it's important for gay men to do safer sex. But it's the gay male community itself which has been really successful in changing sexual practice and educating gay men. And I'm not interested in anyone telling lesbians and everybody else that they ought to do safer sex. That's not to say that sexually active heterosexuals aren't at risk, and although I don't believe lesbian sexual transmission is very likely, I may be proved wrong. Surely what we ought to be trying to do is to create different forms of relationships where there is real trust and honesty. If we had that basis, we wouldn't be having over the top discussions about safer sex - that discussion would be so much more integrated into our relationships, and so much more normalized.

I am surprised by some of my very sexually active heterosexual patients who have many more than one partner and who don't practise safer sex. If I were heterosexual and sexually active like that I would definitely practise safer sex. Somewhere the approach is wrong. Of course in a general sense gay men 'ought' to practise safer sex. I know lesbians who talk about safer sex but they don't practise it. Whatever one does with ones' girlfriend (who might have slept with an intravenous drug 'abuser' five years ago, one year ago, or yesterday), I don't think there's a huge problem of transmission through oral sex or any other lesbian sexual practice, but of course no one can be 100 per cent certain because our knowledge of HIV is so limited and changing.

When I was first sexually active at fifteen or sixteen there was an onslaught of health education about gonorrhoea and syphilis. Everyone I knew was obsessed with it and running off to the VD clinic every two weeks in case they had it. These days there is no effective health education but I'm sure there are plenty of the same STDs around. I see patients who have gonorrhoea or have had it fairly recently. This can be explained partly by cuts in health education budgets. But also there is no sense of urgency about STDs despite there being much more likelihood of being infected by gonorrhoea or warts than HIV. Why isn't it all incorporated into general sex education so that everyone is aware of the whole range of risks, and everyone knows how to use condoms and does so accordingly.

I should get down to describing briefly what classical naturopathy is: it's about using the body's own resources and promoting the body's own ability to be well, keep well, and stay well. Since everybody has to eat, it's based principally around diet - in other words a diet applied to whatever problem you happen to have. If you have asthma, for instance, you stop eating mucous producing foods. For your average, tired, run down person, I would recommend a general, reasonable, good diet which contains lots of fresh fruit and vegetables, whole grains and enough protein. Enough protein means a couple of the following a day: yogurt, fish, eggs, cheese, or meat. Protein is a problem in this country because so many people have gone to the other side of the fence. People tend to have too much protein or they simply don't have enough. If you suggest to somebody that they eat a little more protein it can make the most miraculous difference; it's amazing. Spending a certain unspecified amount of time off all stimulants like coffee, tea, alcohol, cigarettes - all the things that compromise your immune system - is a good idea for everybody to do from time to time. It gives your body a rest and clears it out. If you're feeling run down or you've just had flu or you have colds every other week, it's a good idea to do all the things I've described, as well as taking some herbs to strengthen your system.

Classical naturopathy is only about diet and about using your body, so it also includes breathing exercises and exercising your body. Many naturopaths use other forms of treatment as well. I use herbal remedies because I think they enhance the body's possibilities of healing. Things like blood cleansing herbs and immune strengthening herbs are very good for someone who, for whatever reason, whether it be glandular fever, HIV illnesses, or anything else, needs strengthening. Someone who is under serious emotional stress can benefit from herbs and nerve tonics. Everybody should have basic access to this sort of information; that's what preventative health education should be about. If people didn't run off and take Beecham's powders every time they thought they had a cold, and let their body take care of itself, they'd probably get better, quicker results and wouldn't get a cold again in two weeks' time. But it's not the kind of approach mainstream health education imparts to people.

I use vitamin B and C for stress down feeling run down with great effect but in general I think that vitamins and mineral supplementation is a capitalist growth industry taking advantage of the boom in so-called alternative health. I see a substantial number of patients who are in a terrible state because they have been taking mega-mineral this or mega-vitamin that and it horrifies me. Ordinary basic vitamins in slightly higher doses than you would normally find in food are a good idea as an extra supplement when you've got flu, are around loads of people who are ill or when you've been visiting somebody in hospital everyday. I think there ought to be legislation but the problem in proposing something like that, in our society, is that the people who do the legislating aren't necessarily the people we want to legislate about anything, let alone health. There are practitioners who I respect who use mega-vitamins but I still don't necessarily like it. People do what they think is best. Homeopaths are horrified by people who use herbs, but it doesn't mean that as I use herbs, I'm maliciously causing my patients damage - even though some homeopaths would think so.

I truly believe there are some very good things about allopathic/Western medicine, and I also believe that about most branches of medicine, whether we're talking about acupuncture, homeopathy, naturopathy, herbalism, or anything else. I would like to see a medical system whose structure incorporated all of these health practices and bodies of knowledge.

Let's look at cancer, although it's more complicated than many other illnesses because people are desperately driven when they've got it so they'll try anything: chemotherapy, radiotherapy, drugs, visualization, the whole lot. But, for example, I think that visualization can complement chemotherapy - you can visualize your chemotherapy going round your body killing off all your bad cancer cells. And with conditions like osteoarthritis or rheumatoid arthritis in younger people, if you follow a diet and take herbs, it can give you more of a sense of your own power and control over your symptoms, and that is very good in helping recovery. Herbs and diet have a very good track record in a stricter treatment sense for those kinds of conditions. But also, everybody has a right to sleep, and if the herbs don't get you to sleep and an anti-inflammatory drug does, then great, have a good night's sleep. It's fine to use the holistic things together with something like the odd anti-inflammatory drug. But if someone is on a regimen of gold injections, the odd cortisone injection, and anti-inflammatory drugs twenty-five times a day, that's a different discussion.

I would never pretend that diet and herbs or any other alternative medicine can cure everything. I've changed my mind about cancer over the past few years. A breast lump, for example, will respond much better if you remove the primary focus, in other words the lump, and then do alternative treatment. There is a much better success rate than if you keep the cancer in there and do the alternative treatment.

I am very suspicious of the use of AZT for people who are HIV positive or have AIDS. I don't see it as a form of genocide which some critics claim it is, but I do think it is seriously damaging and also that a lot of people are making an enormous amount of money out of it. I feel that people (so far primarily gay men) are being used as guinea pigs. If I had AIDS, I'd be hard pushed to take AZT, but I don't have AIDS, so I don't know for sure. Desperation makes you try anything. My main reaction against these toxic drug treatments is firstly the money element - it's capitalism making money out of people's misfortune and that makes me angry, and secondly it's about people being used as guinea pigs. What's going to happen in five or fewer years when AZT is suddenly discovered to have horrendous effects and that knowledge becomes common knowledge? It's like Hormone Replacement Therapy (HRT). Year after year there's a new line on it - one year it's great, the next a study says it's loaded with problems, but the year after, it makes another come back.

Sometimes I feel like I'm not presenting myself as a good example of a naturopath because I have contradictory ideas and don't necessarily offer a neat set of rules for people to follow. I really don't believe that people running around trying to have perfect diets, eating only organic food and spinning in circles trying to get their health together, whether they've got HIV or not, is a good thing. It's bad for your health. That kind of obsession is a reflection of the general state of the world, certainly the general state of the Western world.

As I said previously, I don't think that HIV positive people should necessarily to do anything more than everybody else should to do to keep healthy because if we all reassessed what health means, and how we could genuinely practise prevention in a differently ordered society, with a different government and with more power over our lives, that would help remove the stigma attached to AIDS. Carrying around everyone else's prejudices and fears at the same time that you're carrying the virus can't be good for your health if you are HIV positive.

If HIV could be taken off its pedestal and be like glandular fever or cancer or liver disease it would help everyone. Why can't it be like any other disease that sometimes happens to have tragic results like cancer does or liver damage? Why can't it be seen as part of a spectrum of diseases in an overall view of disease? Then we could begin to get away from the idea that HIV=AIDS=Death. We need a society, a world, which has overcome homophobia and racism and all the other forms of structural inequality which exist, in order for that to be fully realized, but that's what we could all be working towards.

How long have we been having these discussions? On and off for ten years or more. AIDS is a relatively new subject but here we are with the same discussion - it's the politics of health, it's the drug companies, it's the multinational companies, it's the effect of capitalism, racism and sexism on people's lives. All this affects us, it implodes on us and it affects the way we feel about ourselves or what our access to health care might be.

In Britain, Central America, in African countries, or anywhere else, it's the same issues with different specifics. But they've got a new growth industry in AIDS. Death is a growth industry, vitamins are, AZT is, HIV is, AIDS is. When are they going to get off our backs? When are they going to let people be? How much more do they want to control us? We have to begin to take control of our lives.

A TRADITIONAL
CHINESE MEDICAL
APPROACH
TO HIV AND AIDS

LEI ZHOU AN

*Zhou was born in Trinidad in 1958 and
came to England in 1976 to study at the
Rambert Ballet School. She completed
her acupuncture course in 1985 through
the Journal of Chinese Medicine and in
1988 she finished a course in Chinese
herbal medicine taught by Giovanni
Maciocia and Ted Kaptchuk.*

I'M PART OF a fourth generation Chinese family living in the
West Indies. I came to England when I was eighteen to train
as a ballet dancer and until I was twenty-eight my life was
devoted to ballet. But the life of a classical dancer is precari-
ous and in 1980 I began thinking about another career. I come
from a medical background and was always drawn to medicine, but I was equally interested in Chinese philosophy and
the Chinese way of being. I lived with an aunt in China for
six months in 1981 and it was at that point that I decided to
study Chinese medicine. On my return to England I started
studying, first acupuncture, and then Chinese herbs - all of which
took about three years to complete.

During the course of my studies I became more and more

interested in AIDS, primarily because as a ballet dancer I had many gay friends and the dramatic and drastic changes in their lives shocked me. Of course I had heard about AIDS and HIV; I'd been in New York in the early 1980s when the epidemic first hit America and seen the first waves of hysteria it created. But it wasn't until I started studying Chinese medicine that I decided to try to understand more about it. I got in contact with a London-based AIDS organization and was involved in some of their support groups before they had proper premises or services, but I still wanted to work somewhere which had clinical experience of treating HIV positive people and people with AIDS. I found my way to New York City's Lincoln Hospital, and a clinic which specialized in treating substance abuse. Dr Michael Smith has been running the clinic for almost fifteen years and it is now a model for alcohol and drug abuse de-toxification programmes all over America and the world. At the beginning of the AIDS crisis people turned up there for help, so now they have over eight years' experience of treating people with the virus.

I returned to England determined to put my experiences into practice here. I wrote to all sorts of places, including the World Health Organization, but nothing materialized. I was still registered as an acupuncturist with the AIDS organization I was originally involved with and eventually someone there rang to ask if I could treat a client who was requesting acupuncture. That's how it began - my list of patients grew and now I have a full quota of patients and a waiting list. Two years ago I wasn't treating any women but now I see between three and eight women each week. Altogether I treat between fifteen to twenty people a week on a one-to-one basis. Acupuncture is part of a range of complementary therapies offered there, including massage, aromatherapy, reflexology, homeopathy, hypnotherapy and art therapy.

People who decide they want to take herbs have to get them paid for by a health authority or have some money stashed away to pay for them. This is a pity, because even if someone is having acupuncture, herbs, taken on a daily basis, can stabilize and improve their quality of life. When the two methods are combined it's very combustible because you're treating on two different but complementary levels or wavelengths.

If herbs are taken in the traditional Chinese way, which is how I prefer to administer them, they need to be cooked and the cost varies between approximately £2.50 and £3.50 a packet with each packet lasting about one or two days. For most people that's a lot of money. If someone needs herbs in pill form it works out a lot cheaper but it's still a financial burden. In general a patient never needs more than four or five bottles for a course of treatment. Thankfully, I've found that most people I'm treating who are receiving benefits are able to get their herbs paid for.

Some HIV positive people come to me with no hope; the most they think they can get out of the treatment is to feel better in themselves, to feel less stressed and more relaxed. Others come to me as a last hope, which is quite an expectation to handle. One of my tasks is to make them realize that hope resides within themselves, not in anyone else.

I start off on a very practical, down-to-earth, medical level. I take name, place of residence, date of birth, and when the person was diagnosed. I ask what medications he or she is on and what Western medical diagnosis has been made. Has the person got an opportunistic infection? After I get all the 'serious' medical bits finished with, I use a traditional Chinese medical method for eliciting information which is the same for anyone whether they're HIV positive or not, whether they've got pre-menstrual tension or feel hot or cold - whatever. I form a picture from the tongue and pulses to help me make the diagnosis I need as an acupuncturist and herbalist. The traditional Chinese diagnosis is the main tool I use in treatment; all the other things that have been happening to a person are added on and used to support of my understanding of the situation. It's possible to use Chinese medicine to treat people without knowing the Western diagnosis, including HIV. However, a

Western diagnosis and treatment means that the patient is likely to be on Western drugs and that is important for me to know.

Next I ask what the person wants to get out of my treatment. Within Chinese medicine, we have two aspects which we assimilate in order to treat. One is the root cause, called Ben, and the other, Biao, is the manifestation - you might call it symptoms. The patients I see are staying for a short time, usually two weeks, and they require treatment which is primarily symptomatic because I see them once or twice or at most four times, and then they go home. I have to gear myself up to figuring out what I can do more or less immediately to help someone. What is it that's really bothering them? If they are vomiting, I treat them for vomiting; I take the same approach for diarrhoea, an awful cough and tickly throat, chills and sweats, stress and inability to settle or sleep at night. I am forced to treat symptomatically because I'm not seeing them on a long-term basis. They want to benefit from one treatment and most times they do, but it's difficult to work in that framework. If you've ever gone to an acupuncturist you know the first thing they tell you is that one treatment is not enough and that the basis of our work is long-term. Most acupuncturists see people on an out-patient basis; they're not carrying out treatment in a hospital, and they're usually not treating them in an acute stage of a chronic or potentially terminal illness.

When you know you will be seeing a patient for a few weeks, you have to change your approach completely but in fact the effects of short-term treatment surprise me each time. Of course it varies to a certain extent; there are times when you make no impact at all. But on the whole the minimum it does is relax the person, make them feel more at ease with themselves, and able to ask for help or be in touch with what is really going on in themselves. In some very acute cases it can help the person be more at peace, to let go and die peacefully. Sometimes it helps them be more lucid so they can have a conversation with their loved ones. With others, it gives them more energy and motivation and they realize it's not the end and they have life left to live.

Having an interaction with someone who can really hear what is being said is important. I'm not trying to suppress their illness with another drug. At times it is difficult to work in this way when there are other practitioners who don't see the patient in the way I do as a traditional Chinese medical practitioner, and who may be working inadvertently against my aims. Everyone is trying to give the patient as much support as they can, but many people, even medical practitioners (myself included), aren't always aware of why certain things are going on. For instance, of course people who are very ill may have diarrhoea or incontinence. Why? Because they're scared shitless about what they fear is going to happen to them. Of course they may come down with diarrhoea and vomiting if they're taking a toxic cocktail of drugs or have Cryptosporidium, a severe bowel infection.

People come to see me who are on many different drugs: 'recreational' ones and the legal drugs used to treat AIDS such as AZT. No one knows exactly what AZT does, and although I feel it is too soon to arrive at any clinical judgement about it, as a practitioner of traditional Chinese medicine, I can see that it interferes with the healthy balance of what we call Qi blood Yin and Yang. The same can be said of many other drugs being used specifically to treat HIV and AIDS. And then there are all the other drugs people are taking such as anti-biotics, anti-nausea, anti-diarrhoea, and anti-depressant pills. I don't dismiss Western medicine, although I am suspicious of it and I know that desperate people will do desperate things.

If people working in different disciplines can work together, they can try to complement each other. What do we want to do if someone has nausea? We want to eliminate it, but at the same time we want the person to take the medicine prescribed for their HIV virus. What if the medicine is causing the nausea? Sometimes you can find a way: perhaps you can use Chinese medicine to alleviate the nausea. In China, the health system often combines different approaches. For example, for a cancer patient they might combine chemotherapy and radiotherapy treatment with Chinese herbs and acupuncture. The herbs and acupuncture may make it possible to reduce the amount of Western drugs and at the same time enhance the patient's ability to effectively absorb them. As well, because of their own properties, the Chinese herbs are helping the patient's condition.

One of the main reasons why Western medicine misses the mark is its inability to get its drugs only to where they're needed. That is where Chinese herbs in particular, and acupuncture and Chinese medicine as a whole, are superior. With herbal medicine, for instance, if we want to help the liver we can send something directly to the liver. Each herb works on meridians, the same way that acupuncture does, so we can direct herbs to a particular part of the body, and to a particular organ to receive its medicine. This explains why Chinese doses are so low. Western medicine hasn't a clue how to direct its herbs or drugs to the injured or affected organ, so it simply floods the body. It's one of the reasons their doses tend to be so high. Recently science has been able to engineer some Western drugs into a targeted area. But this has happened only within the last five or so years. Chinese medicine has been targeting its herbs for the past thousand years or so. Western medicine sometimes uses natural herbs, but only a specific part of the herb which is extracted and purified and only then used as a medicine. In fact this process kills the potency of the medicine. In Chinese herb medicine we use whole parts of the plant, whether it's root, leaf, stem, berry, or bark. If there is a harmful effect in a herb, it often contains its own antidote if taken in its whole form. If we are giving a herb which may have a harmful effect, we give another one which counteracts that possibility. We tend to give a combination of herbs to achieve a unified effect.

Chinese herbs are no more or less powerful than acupuncture. Acupuncture works on one wavelength, herbs work on another. I describe a patient as a landscape: there is a river in the landscape which is the pulses. When you feel the pulses, you sense the quantity and quality of the water in the landscape. When something is missing you put back some nourishment. One way this is achieved is through the liquid herbal form where it goes through all the tributaries to fill out the landscape.

Acupuncture could be described as being more like the external forces of the universe affecting the landscape. The two treatments work in different ways even though they are coming from the same source. I tell my patients that the body is like an electrical circuit and the acupuncture needles are like switches in the circuit. We have several circuits on different layers, so the needles switch on, switch off, activate, stimulate, and sedate the different circuits within our body. These circuits need to harmonize, flush out, strengthen, and fortify. When you put the to different approaches together, it's very effective.

I believe that acupuncture is very useful to people who are HIV positive. Only occasionally, if someone is really very ill, have I decided that an acupuncture treatment might weaken more than strengthen. But perhaps the patient is still asking you for help. If you say no, I can't help you, they feel rejected. What I do in that situation is modify my treatment. In a normal treatment the needles are left in between fifteen and thirty minutes. If someone is very ill in a way which I think counter-indicates a full treatment, instead, I use a couple of needles in the ears or a few in the wrists and leave in for about ten minutes. I use moxa in a minimum of cases because most people I see with HIV-related illness are too hot for it. If I'm seeing extreme cold or deficiency or something which needs to be moved then I apply moxa. Moxa is the external application of smouldering herbs, applied either through a burning stick which the practitioner holds near the skin at specific points or through direct application of the smouldering herb to the skin. My preferred method is to put the herbs on the top of the needle and then the heat descends into the specific point. In any method the patient is in control because he or she indicates when it is getting too hot and the heat is immediately removed.

Most of the time I think it is all right to use acupuncture and herbs in conjunction with other holistic practices. Sometimes after acupuncture or massage a person is pretty wiped out and then I wouldn't treat them. I would never treat a haemophiliac with acupuncture. But personally I don't see anything else that counter-indicates what I'm doing. Some homeopaths think that acupuncture and homeopathy don't go together but as far as I'm concerned if someone is having homeopathy, I can still treat them with acupuncture and herbs if they want.

When people are very ill, their digestive systems are extremely weak, and sometimes they literally cannot digest too many potions of any sort. I had one patient who was taking all kinds of herbs, not Chinese ones, and when he started acupuncture he was suffering from a kind of poisoning. I don't think anything should be taken which over-burdens the system. But if Western medicines 'poison' you, that's supposedly okay because they've been prescribed by a doctor. But if an alternative practitioner 'poisons' someone, that's it, she or he could lose their practice. People have to be very careful about who they go to and what they take. When I give herbs to people who are very ill I start them off on a low dose to see how they respond and how well they absorb them. They have to be strong enough to take more. Also some herbs taste horrible - the ones for skin complaints are probably the worst! I spend ages telling people how disgusting they taste before I give them, so when they finally taste the herbs it's not as bad as I made out.

Any differences in how I treat women and men are not to do with being HIV positive, they're to do with being women or men. In other words it isn't the illness itself which determines the diagnosis and treatment, it's who the person is and their lifestyle which informs those things. Many of the women I treat are mothers, and a significant number of them are single, divorced or widowed, so they carry all the concerns for their children. They worry about the future, about what might happen to the children if they became seriously ill, who would look after them?

I don't say to patients that I believe AZT interferes with their natural balance. How would that help someone who is taking it and believes it's helping them? I might discuss it if they've stopped taking AZT, or even if they have never tried it and are happy that way, because in my experience many of the people I see have had bad side-effects from the drug. There are some who gain weight, get better and look good for a while, but with a traditional Chinese medicine diagnosis, and by feeling the pulses, I often see that pathological changes begin to occur. Also, the people I see who are terminally ill are the people who have been taking high doses of AZT and other drugs. But I see a lot of people at an in between stage, people who have stopped taking AZT who are being treated by me with a combination of acupuncture and herbs. I aim to improve their quality of life and to help them fight off any of the other things which are cropping up because of stopping AZT and possibly being in a weak condition.

I believe human beings are the last link in the food chain and that our world is dying because we are systematically destroying it. Somewhere along the line we may have mutated a virus ourselves, creating HIV. In order for human beings to survive we have to learn to survive this virus. We have created it, and I hope I'm right in thinking that just as we learned to survive tuberculosis and syphilis, we will eventually learn to survive HIV. What will determine how we get better is our ability to survive and adapt. The progression and evolution of people ill with HIV diseases has already changed. World-wide we've reached the third or fourth generation of people with HIV. Maybe in another five or six generations of the disease, although many people will be HIV positive, they might not manifest AIDS.

Practising acupuncture and herbalism is a one-to-one experience and therefore I get very involved and develop a relationship with the patient. But it has to be a professional relationship with clear boundaries. Both myself and my patients have to understand that I am only one part of their medical support. I want to encourage them to understand that ultimately they are the ones who should be in control of their well-being, at the same time as recognizing that some of it is not in their control and is beyond finite human comprehension. There are not necessarily any answers, but there is hope and courage once one comes to terms with ones fears. It's often the case that Western medical doctors tell patients they should take AZT or else they will die prematurely. I usually try to help patients slow down the process of sorting out decisions about treatment if they are frantic and desperate. In those conditions it is unlikely anyone will make the right decision for themselves. In the course of my treatment I try to stabilize the patient mentally and help them discover how to be true to themselves and how they want to live their lives. If they want to have a go at taking AZT, then they should go ahead and I will support that decision. If they want to try out Chinese herbs and acupuncture, with a little bit of Western medicine, then I will support that too. The most important thing is that it is their decision. It is one which will affect the quality of the rest of their lives and shouldn't be made when they have two different voices pushing polarized views at them. People make many unclear decisions; is there ever a clear-cut right or wrong? As we say in Chinese, there only is what is, and what isn't isn't. If people realize that they do have a choice then they don't have to be force-fed by Western medicine or by Chinese medicine or any other discipline.

My aim in life is eventually to have my own traditional Chinese Medicine hospital, as well as gaining clinical experience for research. Not necessarily for AIDS only, because I also treat many other conditions such as migraines, fertility and menstrual irregularities. You could walk into a hospital knowing you could have both traditional Chinese medicine and Western medicine supporting you. I think it is the medicine of the twenty-first century. Even though Western medicine can save lives, paradoxically it can harm the patient in the process. Chinese medicine encourages the person to be, as well as treating pathological disease in a very physical way.

Whether you're HIV positive or not, if you are in tune with a Chinese way of thinking about medicine and see an acupuncturist and take herbs, your chances of staying healthy probably outweigh your chances of getting ill. Well, maybe. Who really knows? Karma is karma. I have some HIV positive patients who are taking herbs and acupuncture, and no Western medicine, who have never felt better in their lives. But they are few and far between because in this climate, you have got to be mentally strong and supported, and very secure in who and what you are in order to do that. People who have been dominated by drug abuse are often uncertain of themselves and of their self-worth, so how can they make real choices about their lives? Trauma and insecurity in someone's life may make it difficult to make choices which are so complex. This is not only about being faced with HIV and AIDS, it's cancer or any other life threatening condition. Suddenly life becomes so precious and your emphasis is on it. How you treat yourself and others, how they treat you, are all accented. You don't become a 'better person' because you are ill, but your focus can change and life can have a new meaning.

Anyone who wants to find out more about Traditional Chinese medicine should ring up the Institute of Complementary Medicine and ask for the address of the Registrar of Traditional Chinese Medicine (RTCM). That's a first step. The next best step, or even the best, is by word of mouth. Ask around. You could also approach your local AIDS helpline because they might be gathering information on different forms of treatment and know an acupuncturist. Sometimes a women's centre will have information about acupuncturists or herbalists and some even have women practitioners who see people at the centre. If you are HIV positive or have AIDS remember that you are not alone and that there are trained people to help and inform you, so that you don't feel isolated or abandoned. There is support for you, especially in Britain; people from all over Europe and Africa come to London for their treatment. But there is still so much which needs to be addressed, medically, socially, politically and emotionally. It's just the beginning!

HOUSING NEEDS OF POSITIVE WOMEN

ROZ PENDLEBURY

*Roz Pendlebury has worked in housing
for sixteen years, eight with homeless
women, and four on the housing needs of
people with HIV at the AIDS and
Housing Project. She is an active
member of the UK Declaration of the
Rights of People with HIV and AIDS
working party. Since April 1992 she has
been the general manager of
The Landmark in London.*

I GOT INVOLVED in housing through working at Homeless
Action, a project for housing single homeless women, and that
experience focused me, among other things, on questions of
discrimination and housing. At the time, HIV and AIDS were
largely seen as having to do with gay men, but as a lesbian I
thought about the issue immediately, and realized that discrimination on grounds of sexuality was bound to increase. I went
on to work on policy at the AIDS and Housing Project which
was set up to ensure that a range of housing options were made
available to people with HIV and AIDS.

The project is a very small organization, although it covers
all of England, Scotland and Wales. Our brief includes a mixture of training, mainly for housing organizations, and policy
work, which in practice means developing guidelines for housing

organizations. We advise housing associations, local authorities, and voluntary projects on the steps they need to take in order to make their services open to people with HIV. A lot of our work concentrates on issues of confidentiality, equal opportunities policies and practice, and infection control policies in housing organizations. In our policy work we respond to legislation; for instance, we have been trying to get housing and HIV included in the National Health Service and Community Care Act. As we obtain new information, we present it to agencies such as the Department of Environment and the Housing Corporation, to encourage changes in policy.

More recently, I have been very involved in developing The UK Declaration of Human Rights of People with HIV. General human rights, agreed to by the UK, are not being upheld for people with HIV. Women with HIV have specific problems with diagnosis and treatment and these areas need to be targeted. Housing needs also raise important rights issues.

In training sessions the AIDS and Housing Project often finds it necessary to go through all the basics to do with HIV transmission, even though transmission has absolutely nothing to do with being a housing officer. As one Director of Housing put it, 'There is no risk of HIV transmission at work for housing staff unless they are having sex or taking drugs with the tenants.' But we still have to cover it because many people who attend our training sessions come with a sub-text: they need to work through their own fears about HIV transmission. Unless you address their fears and give them information, they won't take seriously (or even take in) the rest of the training.

It's taken over three years of building a reputation as the experts in the field, to get local authorities and housing associations to take us seriously. When I started the job I had a clear strategy in mind about how to make our organization succeed. At Homeless Action, one problem was that as providers of housing we'd never sponsored basic pieces of research. Because no one had ever properly researched women's homelessness on any scale, it was hard to argue the reality of the hidden homelessness of women. Although everyone who works around homelessness knows that women's hidden homelessness exists, unless you can quote statistics, it's very hard to get any credibility. At the AIDS and Housing Project we have started doing targeted pieces of research, usually focusing on the needs of consumers. For example, we carried out a study of people with HIV which asked about the housing they were in; what they thought their housing needs were; and how their health related to their housing. The study was based in an area of mixed housing tenure, where there was a racially diverse population, because we specifically wanted to include women and black people. The study wasn't large enough to conclude that proportionately women want one thing, or men another, but it was interesting that most of the people in it were in incredibly bad housing. Because they were single, many had been housed in hard-to-let schemes; they had a roof over their heads, but it was of very poor standard and they were stuck with it.

Our findings were that many people had quite limited housing desires: often it boiled down to wanting central heating and a shower. Central heating featured because of all the respiratory problems people with HIV can develop. Also if someone is experiencing weight loss and fevers, they will feel the cold more. Having a shower was another focus, because if someone's weight drops it can be very uncomfortable getting in and out of a bath. As well, if someone is getting night-sweats and perhaps has bad diarrhoea, they want to be able to wash easily and that is helped by being able to step into a shower quickly. Also, modern housing developments, adaptations, or renovations of old property tend to squeeze the bathroom into the smallest possible space, and people with HIV-related illnesses find it hard to manage in such restricted spaces. Major issues around security came up too. After central heating and a shower, people wanted safer locations and better locks.

These are really basic housing desires. Yet a lot of people don't have housing which provides them with these fundamental amenities, or much hope of achieving them. The waiting time for transfers and adaptations is often years. In one London Borough, 40 per cent of people with AIDS die while still in temporary accommodation, waiting to be allocated a permanent flat. It is all too common for people with HIV to be told that unless they are actually ill they can't be rehoused. It's terribly frustrating because anyone who is HIV positive, and well, is aware of the importance of staying healthy, yet housing officials tell them they can't get rehoused until they are ill. It's a catch-22 situation. One of the staggering findings of our survey is that there are many local authorities in the country who won't consider someone with an AIDS diagnosis for rehousing. Even that diagnosis doesn't make them vulnerable under the Homeless Persons' Act unless there are other factors involved. One of the problems the project has faced, is that although it's relatively easy to demonstrate that bad housing is detrimental to good health, it's much more difficult to produce 'hard' evidence that if someone gets rehoused in better housing it helps them to stay healthy.

The Department of Health, and many doctors, say it is impossible to claim that stress increases immune-deficiency. We're not allowed to say that, even though one of the major things people with HIV or AIDS say to us, is that the stress created by living in bad housing is damaging their health. However, at this point, there is no research which directly links the two things.

Home ownership is also an important issue for some people with HIV. We have been looking at mortgage rescue schemes to see how they might apply to people with HIV. One problem with mortgage rescue schemes is that they often have been developed with the elderly in mind, in a situation where over the years people have built up a reasonable amount of equity on their property. They are then able to offset the equity against the cost of reducing the mortgage. Many people with HIV have bought within the last five to seven years when the housing market was high; they haven't built up a lot of equity and so it's more difficult to find a solution which enables them to stay in their house. Because most HIV positive women have never been part of the house-buying market, this is usually not relevant to them.

In relation to preserving HIV positive tenants' confidentiality, our work with service providers concentrates on countering any feelings of obligation they have to inform anyone else about a client's HIV status. We have a surprising number of examples where someone, perhaps with the kindest of motives, breaks confidentiality. For instance, a woman with AIDS is very ill, so the community nurse mentions to her neighbour that she's got AIDS and needs a helping hand. If the woman had cancer the neighbour might be helpful, but since she has AIDS, instead of help she may get 'slag' or 'prostitute' painted on her front door. People have been fire-bombed because they were known, or believed, to have AIDS and that doesn't happen if you have cancer.

As far as women are concerned, local authorities don't monitor, so we just don't know how many of the HIV positive people they have rehoused are women. We also have no idea of the numbers of people who won't approach an authority for housing because they are too worried about disclosing their status.

It would be wonderful if we could get the housing associations we are working with to take on the HIV/AIDS education of their members, but in fact we have enough trouble getting a housing department trained. In a few cases, Glasgow for instance, we have done training with the whole housing department from top to bottom. We have also worked with the London borough of Newham, and in Hounslow, we've been employed as consultants to develop an HIV policy for the housing department, all of which is encouraging. In our survey, no one had done any work with tenants, only one local authority housing department mentioned a consumer organization they communicated with, and only one said, 'We've talked to Body Positive' (an organization for HIV positive people).

It is a terrible uphill struggle, although an obviously necessary one. In many ways it can be seen in the same context as equal opportunity work generally: you have a fantasy that people will suddenly seeing the light and be transformed. But in reality, it's plodding day-to-day work. You do a training session one year and then maybe the next year someone will remember it and come back for more, and then maybe they'll end up with a policy. I've known organizations to take up to three years to develop a policy. Equal opportunities work is long term. It's similar to the issue of confidentiality which is also a new field for housing organizations. Everyone thinks they believe in confidentiality, but it is broken all the time. To give an example, at a community health centre on a housing estate in London, the receptionist blurted out, 'Oh, you're the person with AIDS'. The aftermath of that one small remark was fifteen people having to be moved off the estate by the council. Not, I might add, because they were all HIV positive, but because they were perceived as members of a group which was 'at risk' - in other words for being gay or Black.

People from African countries often are seen as being at risk by virtue of being African - as if they were a monolithic group. Discrimination can be very complex. Someone might be HIV positive but the way in which discrimination is manifested might be homophobia or racism. Perhaps someone doesn't have HIV but happens to be from Uganda or be a gay man but they are assumed to be HIV positive by virtue of their identity.

I think HIV is very similar in a lot of ways to other conditions which affect housing needs. It's a chronic health condition which impacts on those needs. There are some links with cancer and how it used to be seen in the past, when there were fears about its transmission. What makes HIV different is the link with discrimination. HIV is still perceived as something which affects minority or oppressed groups: gay men, drug users, black people. They are seen as 'other' by the so-called mainstream, white, heterosexuals. Marginalization and discrimination then interact with the fact that being HIV positive may lead to chronic illnesses and in some cases death.

In our training we look at how housing managers might deal

with this combination: suppose you have someone who is a drug user, also seriously ill, and in rent arrears. Do you deal with that person in the same way as anyone else in rent arrears? Do you bring in moral overtones which might not have come into play with someone else in similar rent difficulties who wasn't a drug user? Let's face it, a proportion of elderly people in local authority accommodation who have dementia are a hell of a burden to their neighbours. But the same moral dimension is not brought into play with them as with the drug user. We have met a senior officer in a housing authority who said about people with AIDS, 'Why should I help people who have brought this upon themselves?'

People make moral judgements about HIV all the time, a factor which is partially what differentiates it from other health conditions. My personal feeling is that in the current climate people working around housing and HIV/AIDS could make more links with disability campaigns. There are other immune-deficiency conditions and illnesses like sickle-cell anaemia and ME. Some HIV illnesses are chronic infections, not acute ones, so there are very clear links with something like ME. But making these links practical is easier said than done; too often people fall into a competitiveness about housing - instead of campaigning for housing for everyone in need, they want 'their' particular group put at the top of a hierarchy of housing needs.

Housing needs are complex. You only have to think about the process of selection and allocation. People with HIV are often stereotyped as being single, and single people are often given hard-to-let accommodation. People with HIV might be accepted as homeless but will still get offered hard-to-let type accommodation because that is what the authorities give to single people. But it is not appropriate to their needs. In any case, not all HIV positive people, and particularly women, are single. There are huge issues about bed and breakfast accommodation: much evidence indicates that living in bed and breakfast accommodation has a detrimental health effect. Research projects which have focused on women and children in bed and breakfasts show a higher level of mortality and evidence of increased low level mental illness.

Women who are HIV positive or have AIDS face all the same housing problems that other women face, plus their specific needs. Hidden homelessness is the main issue for women. Previous to the AIDS epidemic, a struggle was underway to gain recognition that homelessness is broader than rooflessness. But under the present administration the tendency is more and more to define homelessness as rooflessness - people who are living on the streets. Most women who are homeless are sleeping on other people's floors; sometimes they end up in relationships in order to get housed. The danger for women of street homelessness is much greater than for men. It is not just physical danger: sexual harassment is a continuous possibility. Within the homeless population, women's homelessness isn't visible; within that, women with HIV become doubly invisible. It happens again and again with women and HIV: you are disadvantaged as a women, and then the HIV comes on top of that.

The AIDS and Housing Project is also concerned about the relationship between homelessness and risk behaviour. Research from here and the United States shows that being homeless encourages people into risk-taking. Homelessness creates a feeling of hopelessness and a lack of self-worth, a feeling of not being valued by society. The temptation to take drugs in order to forget, have sex for warmth and intimacy, or for money, is high. When self-esteem is low and privacy limited, the possibility of doing these things safely is limited.

Women refugees face their own specific problems around HIV. We know HIV exists in some refugee communities, but people from these communities are terrified to approach housing authorities. For a start, they may not understand the way the housing system works and not have access to good advice. There are people trying to get refugee status who are positive and, understandably, they may have anxieties about making a demand on a housing service. If they reveal their positive status will it affect their immigration status, or get them kicked out of the country? For these people, isolation is a problem, because a lot of the refugee communities are very small and being known to be HIV positive in the community can bring discrimination in its wake. Often there is literally no one a refugee woman can talk to. Blackliners were rung by a woman who wouldn't come to their office, preferring to meet in a cafe to get advice about a housing problem, because of her fear of being found out. If you have only got a small community in this country, the dangers of losing that can be unbearable. We have heard about a consultant who had to manage the hospital's appointment system extremely carefully so it was possible to see several people from the same community and maintain confidentiality. It is that sort of practical situation we are dealing with. I knew of a woman, her husband, and all the children who were HIV positive and they would not go to the local authority for help with housing because they felt it would affect their immigration status. And who can say with any certainty that it wouldn't? Luckily, there is now a woman housing adviser at the Terence Higgins Trust, and she can help with many of these problems.

What I am saying over and over again is that there are specifics attached to an HIV positive status, but this society's structures of oppression and exploitation rebound on that status and exacerbate its effects. That is why we all have to work so hard to bring to light all the issues which effect health and well-being.

LEGAL CONCERNS
OF WOMEN WITH
HIV OR AIDS

SIMMY VIINIKKA

*Simmy Viinikka is a solicitor with a
background in child care and family law.
She has worked in both private practice
and local government and has been
employed at the Terrence Higgins Trust
for eighteen months. She has been a
volunteer and management committee
member of a number of women's
organizations including two rape crisis
centres and a women's aid refuge.*

I AM EMPLOYED at the Terrence Higgins Trust to do legal
work for people affected by HIV and AIDS. About a fifth of
my clients are women and the rest men, which probably reflects
the reality of HIV in England at the moment. I have found that
the legal problems of the women I see are a reflection both of
the problems experienced by women in society generally and
of those experienced by men with HIV. My female clients tend
to be poorer, more socially disadvantaged, and are more likely
to be black than the men I see, and their problems are exacer-
bated by these factors.

I see a number of women who have recently come from
African countries. Some are political refugees, others have come

here to get married, to study or to take up employment and then they discover they are HIV positive. They have all the problems of racism, in addition to their HIV status. Some women have a drug history which is socially and economically stigmatizing. I also give advice, particularly on the telephone, to many women who may be perceived more as 'pillars of society', women married to men with haemophilia or who, perhaps, had a blood transfusion in the early 1980s, or who are considering adopting a child with HIV. Such women can be very isolated in different parts of the country, lacking in support, and very concerned about confidentiality.

Women who are HIV positive are sometimes less assertive than men in a similar situation. I suspect that they may not have such a strong sense of their rights, or know where to go to get help, advice or support. Until recently, many HIV specific agencies were geared to the needs of white, gay men which has meant that women who may, in any event, be more isolated, either in the suburbs of London or small towns elsewhere, are excluded. They may be more likely to get their support through traditional means, such as their local Social Services department.

I do not give advice on welfare rights and housing at The Terrence Higgins Trust because we have an excellent department for this, but I believe that money and housing are the key essentials that people with HIV need. I give legal advice on a range of issues such as wills, immigration, insurance, medical complaints, family law, breaches of confidence, property disputes and so on.

People who are diagnosed as negative, or who have not been tested, come to us for help on a number of issues. For example, someone in their family may be positive, or someone may have died or they may be being discriminated against because it is assumed that they are positive. That is, of course, a central issue for gay men because of the prejudice which equates AIDS with gay men. It is not generally expected that women will be HIV positive; this relative invisibility in relation to HIV can be double-sided for women.

I do family work for both men and women. I try to help parents with decision-making regarding who is going to look after their children if they become ill, or die. I know of many instances where a father has been diagnosed with HIV has been stopped from seeing his children. In some cases, court proceedings have been issued but, so far, we have been able to resolve these disputes without a court hearing. By being able to liaise with other departments of the Trust and outside agencies, I am better placed than most solicitors in private practice to try to resolve family disputes by extra-legal means. For example, in some cases a parent may be denying contact with the children because they are very angry about how their spouse became positive and they also may have very little information about transmission of the virus and consequently have imprecise notions about the danger to their children. The Trust is able to help by offering services such as accurate and up-to-date health information and counselling. We have a family support group and also work very closely with the Barnardo's Positive Options project which has been able to offer very constructive intervention in a number of cases.

I spend a great deal of my time preparing wills for people with HIV or AIDS. Many people anticipate that preparing a will may be daunting and distressing, and for that reason put it off. I think it is best for everyone to make a will when they are fit and healthy. Many women with children find the task extremely painful because they need to confront the possibility that they may have to arrange for someone other than themselves to bring up their children in the future. Among the women I see there are many different cultural attitudes to talking about death, funerals and wills and it is important to have some sensitivity in recognizing these.

Many women are extremely concerned about confidentiality. This is a subject about which I have ambivalent feelings. On the one hand, confidentiality is officially protected in many different ways. For example, the Department of Social Services (DSS) and many other government departments are under an obligation of confidentiality, doctors and lawyers are bound by their own professional rules of confidentiality, and information given to STD clinics is protected by law. Moreover, there is a 'common law' of confidentiality enforced by the courts. So there actually exists quite a high legal duty of confidence, the extent of which most people are unaware. On the other hand, understandably, many people's fears are not allayed by these official policies and provisions. For instance, medical information is protected, but files are still trolleyed around and many people in the daily course of their work are entitled to go through these files. Also, the very act of enforcing one's right to confidentiality may result in making the issue more public. For example, there are many cases in which I am not able effectively to represent someone because it would involve contacting the other party on Terrence Higgins Trust headed paper. Nevertheless, I think it is important that people, in so far as it is possible, do not become paralysed and disempowered by a perceived need for secrecy. It should be remembered that any employee in any job who has access to confidential information will be aware that a breach of confidentiality could result in the loss of their job.

The problem is that while there is no obligation to tell anyone one's HIV status, without such disclosure it may not be possible to obtain certain facilities, such as priority treatment in relation to housing or social services provision. Another example involves the immigration service. Many people are fearful of telling the Home Office that they are HIV positive. There is no need to disclose this information, but if they have no other grounds to stay in this country, they might be advised to seek leave to remain on exceptional compassionate grounds which would involve disclosure of their HIV status. I see my role as explaining to people their choices and the possible consequences that might result, but ultimately the decision to disclose one's status is a matter for each individual.

The practical issues which people with HIV need to consider

depend on their situation. It is a good idea for women who are working to think about their pension provision, and whether early retirement on medical grounds might be a future option for them. A woman will also want to gauge how sympathetic her employer might be if she told him or her, or they came to know of her HIV status. Whether or not a woman is at present in employment, it is a good idea to look at the range of welfare benefits which she might be able to obtain, either now or in the future. If a woman has children, the sooner she is able realistically to consider the options for their care if she becomes ill, the better. Women with and without children will want to consider what their local services department might be able to offer them in terms of support, whether this be a home-help or the provision of a telephone. Making a will can be a lot simpler than it sounds, and this will make clear who will be responsible for arranging a funeral, who is to inherit any property and who is able to take care of any children. At the same time it may be advisable to sign an enduring power of attorney which appoints a friend or relative to take financial decisions on your behalf.

I am involved in a new initiative at the Trust to formulate and promote a Living Will for use by people with HIV. Living Wills are not common in this country but are widely used in the USA and in many European countries. Our Living Will is designed to enable people with HIV to state in advance their wishes regarding health care at the end of life and to appoint someone to participate in medical decisions on their behalf if they become unable to do so. This is potentially an exciting project, although I am aware that for some people with HIV who lack basic necessities, such as a roof over their head, the making of a Living Will involving philosophical decisions about the sort of medical treatment they might want at the end of life may be fairly low down in their list of priorities.

Anyone affected by HIV can contact the THT Advice Centre, or Immunity, another AIDS organization, for legal advice. However, Immunity is not able to take on family work at present, so they refer it here. I am also the only woman solicitor doing legal work for people with HIV, at the moment, so I see those who particularly want to see a woman. We are able to advise anyone in the country, but do not usually travel outside London. I make regular home and hospital visits to people within the London area who are not well enough to come and see me at my office. I help clients outside London to try to locate a sympathetic local solicitor or advice bureau. I spend much time doing emergency work such as wills, for people who are really very sick.

The drawback, generally, of the legal system is that it can be slow. One has to wait, firstly to get legal aid, secondly to get a court date, and so on. The client might be getting more and more unwell in the meantime. The delay and resulting stress caused to people with HIV, together with fears about their confidentiality can, in my opinion, mean that they are in practice, often denied a traditional legal remedy. For these reasons I think it is very important to consider other options to resolving a dispute, some of which I have already outlined.

One of the major things which has to change is the attitude of people generally to HIV. In the long-term I don't think the answer is to bolster up secrecy. The answer must be to make it acceptable to say one is HIV positive, in the same way that it is possible to talk about any other chronic and potentially life-threatening condition. Unfortunately, we are clearly still a long way from this goal and the concern about confidentiality, expressed particularly by women with children, must be respected.

PREGNANCY, HIV
AND WOMEN

SUE O'SULLIVAN

*Sue O'Sullivan has written elsewhere in
this book about sexuality, and is an
editor of Positively Women. This
chapter was written after discussion with
Dr Mary Hepburn*.*

ON DISCOVERING THEIR positive HIV status many women
are told in no uncertain terms that they must never become
pregnant. It is heavily implied that pregnancy would be irresponsible on at least three counts: the risk of giving birth to a
baby who may eventually turn out to be HIV positive; the risk
that a pregnancy will have an adverse effect on the health of a
positive mother; and the possibility that the mother will become
ill and die, leaving a young child, positive or not, without a
mother.

For many women who want to have a child, or hope to have
more, this message can be one of the most devastating pieces
of advice they are given. Time after time, positive women tell
of the distress it has caused them.

In fact, the issues pertaining to HIV and pregnancy are not
so clear-cut. Women living with HIV need supportive help,
and relevant non-judgemental information and counselling about
pregnancy and HIV, in order to make their own decisions about
whether or not to consider having a baby. They need the same
input if they discover they are already pregnant, whether before or after they find out they are positive.

Having a child involves much more than the purely physical. Expectations and meanings attached to motherhood vary in different groups of women, influenced, for instance, by culture and class, and economics. Ironically, in this society, women who choose not to have children are often put under enormous pressure to justify their decision by those who view motherhood as women's 'natural' and most fulfilling role. Positive women find themselves under the opposite pressure: don't have children, that would be selfish and irresponsible. Also, it is interesting that many opponents of abortion suddenly forget their rigid stance when confronted with the possibility of positive women having children. Indeed, whatever their position on abortion, many professionals dealing with pregnant HIV positive women, urge them to have abortions without offering a serious, open-ended discussion about choice.

Studies now appear to make it clear that pregnancy will have no adverse effect on an asymptomatic HIV positive woman's HIV infection. In other words, if someone is HIV positive and well, a pregnancy will not result in any acceleration of her HIV infection.

Studies also suggest that a woman's HIV positive status will not adversely affect a pregnancy. In other words, being positive does not, in itself, prevent the development of a healthy fetus, or a normal new-born baby, with the possible exception that HIV may be transmitted to the fetus. Of course that exception is a serious one, and may be the major reason why a woman who is positive and considering pregnancy, or who is already pregnant, will decide not to have a child. The decision, however, is not as straightforward as women have often been led to believe.

How does the possible transmission of HIV to the fetus happen? In the first place, it is important to have a basic understanding of the relationship of the fetus to the mother. Sometimes people get confused about the mother's and the fetus' blood systems. They know that in the womb, the growing baby is being nourished by the mother, and imagine that her blood flows through the baby's body. In fact, the mother's blood system is entirely separate from the baby's. There is no mixing of their blood. The two blood systems exist side by side, separated by a membrane. Some things can pass through the barrier of the membrane, such as the mother's antibodies. All babies are born with their mother's antibodies. Although HIV can pass through the membrane, in the majority of cases it does not.

When the baby of a positive woman is born, it will usually test HIV positive because it has the mother's antibodies. Very occasionally a baby will test negative at birth and later become positive, but this is exceptional. For the majority of babies born to positive women, it takes approximately eighteen months to two years until tests can determine whether or not the toddler is really HIV positive or negative.

There are different predictions on the numbers of babies of positive women who will be positive themselves. They vary between one in eight, to one in two. New studies throw up new numbers. Clearly there is a risk, but one which no one is certain about at this point. As with so much else about AIDS, we do not have certain answers to the questions people most want some certainty around.

What are the issues which HIV positive women will want to take into account when and if they are considering having a baby? These are many and have their origins in different places. Some issues originate with women themselves: 'How can I best make this decision for myself and for any child I might have?' 'How can I weigh up the situation?' Other issues, which will affect positive women, appear to originate with the professionals they will come in contact with, most often doctors and social workers, or to have their roots in a public lack of knowledge or support of people living with HIV.

For women who do not know their HIV status, questions arise about HIV screening. How would a positive result influence their attitude towards a pregnancy? How would others react, such as partners, family, friends or health care practitioners? Would a positive result mean pressure to terminate a pregnancy? Women who believe that there could be a possibility that they are positive, perhaps because of their own, or their partner's drug use, or because of their partner's bi-sexuality, may be put off testing for HIV if they fear negative attitudes and pressure. Women who are drug users may be afraid of admitting this, for fear of losing custody of their children. Testing for HIV should never be undertaken without counselling, whatever the perceived risk of infection is by either the woman or the medical profession. In relation to pregnancy, testing should always be carried out for the benefit of the woman, never as a supposed means of protection of others.

For example, in England and particularly in Scotland, HIV infection in women is often related to intravenous drug use, either by the woman herself, or by her partner. Too often, it is still the case that someone who is HIV positive and/or a current or ex-drug user, or the partner of someone who is, is considered a 'bad' person, certainly not fit to be a mother. However, as Dr Mary Hepburn, who has been providing a service for women with or at risk of HIV infection in Scotland says, 'In our experience in Glasgow, drug use and child care are not incompatible.' What is important in relation to children, is that a woman can achieve a stable lifestyle and be a responsible parent.

Dr Hepburn goes on to describe the issues which affect HIV positive women having babies, and insists that these are as often and as importantly, social, economic, cultural, and religious. Drugs may be a problem for some women, but other worries may include 'housing, attitudes of neighbours, difficulties with or lack of employment, and the health, education and future of existing children - in addition to concerns about their own health and fears surrounding the child as yet unborn.'

If a positive woman is getting purely medical advice on pregnancy, social problems may not be sympathetically addressed, nor practical advice and information available. If there are fears about child custody, and these are not the figments of women's imaginations, then some women may decide it is too risky to talk openly about having a baby, or may even decide not to use the service which is available because it is perceived as hostile and not meeting her needs.

When considering the risk of transmitting HIV to an unborn child, or of adversely affecting the positive mother's own health, it is important to put things into perspective. As Dr Hepburn says, 'It is worth noting here that women with other conditions which reduce life expectancy are less likely to receive such advice. Furthermore, the risk of maternal transmission of HIV to the baby is no worse and, in fact, better than for many other congenitally transmitted conditions.'

Many women have contradictory feelings about birth-control, pregnancy and abortion. Making decisions and putting them into practice does not necessarily mean that the contradictory feelings have disappeared. If a positive woman decides to have a baby, she may well continue to ask herself if she has made the right decision and worry about the risks to the baby. If she decides not to have a child, or if pregnant, to have an abortion, she may well continue to have feelings of ambivalence and regret. All these feelings are common among women, positive or not. But if the decision, whatever it is, has come out of her own weighing up of the pros and cons, then ambivalences can be woven into the overall tapestry of her life. They are part of her decision, her control over her own life. Again Dr Hepburn puts it well: 'Counselling and advice are not synonymous; although one can speculate on what the ultimate risk to the fetus will be, the risk itself is not a matter of opinion; the acceptability of the risk, however, is entirely a matter of opinion and will vary from one individual to another. No one can make a decision about the acceptability of that risk except the individual woman concerned, and the woman should be *counselled* to allow her to make the decision which she feels is right for her and should not be *advised* to act in the way which health care staff feel is appropriate.'

Once a positive woman has decided to get pregnant, or to continue with a pregnancy, the most important thing is for her to stay as healthy as possible, in the way any other woman considering pregnancy would. There are differences of opinion on whether or not drug treatment for HIV, especially with AZT, should continue or be started during pregnancy. Whatever the opinions are on this, following as good a diet as possible, getting plenty of rest, and remaining physically active, are good guidelines for the woman trying to get pregnant, and the pregnant woman.

Anyone who has had a child knows how exhausting a newborn baby can be, so it is not only the effects of HIV on pregnancy which a positive woman will want to think about. Are there friends and services which can offer practical assistance once the baby is born? Will a partner be supportive? Are money worries going to be an ever present concern? How can they be relieved? All these questions deserve consideration. If services for positive women could house more than the medical under one roof, both social services and medical services could back each other up and make life a lot easier for most women.

Once a woman is pregnant and wants to be, as far as possible every single bit of excitement and happiness should be nurtured. Risks have been weighed up. The possibility of having a positive child has been contemplated and the mother-to-be has decided, yes, I can cope with that possibility. Of course she will hope that her child is not HIV positive, but her baby is wanted, whatever happens. If she hasn't been able to see that possibility in her future, she hopefully has been able to make the equally justifiable decision not to have a child, or to have an abortion.

Positive women are no different from other women, except for the impact the virus has on them. It would be silly to think that every positive woman who has a child ends up enjoying every single moment of motherhood. Most mothers (and fathers) have times (and the nights are somehow the worst) of wondering whether they can cope or not. Just because a positive woman has, through circumstances, been forced to be much more self-conscious about the decision to have a baby, doesn't mean she has to pretend to be a blissful mum, twenty-four hours a day. In a perfect world, all mothers would get more practical and emotional support than they do at present. Positive mothers have the extra burden of coping with the virus. Services must be fought for which meet their needs as positive women, as mothers, and as people who have different economic, social, cultural, and emotional needs.

Because the positive woman cannot know for quite a while if her child will be positive or not, there is every reason in the world to concentrate on the ordinary/extraordinary experiences of being a mother, as any other mother would do. The statistics of HIV risk to the baby are relevant when a woman is deciding whether or not to have a child. Once the baby is born, they are irrelevant. The most important thing then is to treat the baby as normal and healthy.

What positive women need most in relation to questions about pregnancy is access to counselling which is not moralistic and judgemental. They want a chance to take in information, digest it, come up with new questions, take in new information, and to explore fully their own feelings and emotions. They will do so in the context of the rest of their lives. They will be faced with difficult decisions, and possibly the necessity for coping with all sorts of changes in their lives. They will do so in a society which often treats women as second-class citizens, and HIV positive women as morally reprehensible and stigmatized. Women, at different times, and in different situations, have had to fight for the right to make choices to have children and the choice to remain childless, or to have an abortion. All of these decisions should come from women themselves, in light of their understanding of their own realities.

* Hepburn, Mary. 'Obstetrics, Women and Drug Use in the Context of HIV' from *Women, HIV, Drugs : Practical Issues,* ed. Shiela Henderson, Institute for the Study of Drug Dependants, London, 1990, pp 45-51.

THINKING ABOUT
THE ISSUES

HOPE MASSIAH

*Hope is twenty-nine, was born in
Barbados, came to England in 1969, and
has been a south Londoner ever since.*

I HAVE BEEN working at Positively Women since June 1991.
I started life as a maths teacher, but since 1987 I've been doing
training research and developmental work (whatever that means)
around black, women's and lesbian and gay issues. It is important to me to work on issues I feel strongly about, so working
around HIV feels like a natural progression. Previously I worked
as an Equalities Officer for Haringey council, but since racism,
sexism, heterosexism and all the other 'isms' have been almost
totally eradicated (or so they seem to think), they decided to
make drastic cuts to the Equalities Unit. I managed to jump
before I was pushed.

In terms of my awareness around HIV, I was pretty slow
on the uptake. I was aware, but when it came to actually thinking it through for myself, it took a long while. When the
information about HIV started to reach me, there wasn't anything in it about how it might affect lesbians. I remember watching a television programme in which they talked about homosexuals and heterosexuals and it was obvious that homosexuals meant men. Lesbians didn't feature in any of the statistics, not even as a zero, or a little footnote indicating that nothing was known about lesbians and HIV. We didn't exist. Of
course I was aware of HIV 'out there', and I knew it was a bad

thing, but it wasn't affecting me personally. No one was telling me I ought to change my life - it was as if there was this frightening epidemic which had nothing to do with me in terms of my sexuality, so my first reaction was phew, thank god, what a relief I don't have to think about this in my own life. It wasn't a fully conscious thought process; I think I was unconsciously relieved that I didn't have to change very dramatically. I worried a bit about whether I might be HIV positive because I'd slept with men less than ten years ago and I'm the sort of person who wonders about every illness that comes along.

Then while I was working in Haringey I got involved in a lesbians and HIV group which was made up of women working around HIV, and we quickly realized we had different expectations of the group. Some of the women worked in care providing roles and their expectations were different from those of us who wanted to concentrate more on general health education for lesbians. We split into two separate groups and I am now part of the health education one; we're working towards running workshops on HIV for lesbians. Part of the process of setting this up has been to think about what we wanted to deal with - did we want to change lesbians' sexual behaviour or did we want them to more fully understand what the deal was so they could then decide whether they wanted to change their behaviour? Personally I think it's more about enabling people be aware of what the situation is as far as we know. The fact is that, no, there are not many lesbians who are HIV positive through sexual contact, but there are a few cases where it seems fairly likely to have happened through sex, and we should let women know that. It's tough to say to lesbians that every time you have oral sex you have to use a dental dam. It's tough for me, because I'm unsure about it myself and to be able to give a clear message to others I have to be pretty confident it's necessary. Right now there is very contradictory advice around: on the one hand there are those who say that all lesbians should be using dental dams, and on the other there are many leaflets advising heterosexuals that oral sex is fine and safe unless the woman is having her period.

Does anyone really think that lesbians aren't going to read the oral-sex-is-okay leaflets, or that maybe they think the virus can tell the difference between lesbians and heterosexuals having oral sex! Either it's all right, or it isn't, or it's safer than other forms of sex, or no one really knows. Do you need to protect yourself or your partner with a dental dam all the time or don't you? I certainly don't want health educationalists or concerned lesbians telling us to use dental dams just to give lesbians something to do in the epidemic. Sometimes I feel pretty sure I don't need to use a dental dam all the time, because the consensus seems to be that oral sex is okay for heterosexuals, so why shouldn't it be for lesbians? However, and it's a big however, I'm untested, I don't know my HIV status. Does that mean that if I were in a relationship with a woman who knew she was HIV positive, that I'd feel perfectly all right not using a dental dam? It's a good question to ask yourself. If you want to use a dental dam because you know someone is positive, or you are, aren't you being irrational if you think it's okay not to, when you don't know?

I'm not saying that I think everyone should rush out and be tested. But it does make me think that maybe we don't think lesbian oral sex is that safe after all, if we want to use a dental dam when we think someone might be, or is, positive. Therefore maybe there is a part of me, like other people, which is assuming the person I sleep with isn't positive.

There are a lot of lesbians working around HIV but not directly about anything to do with lesbians. To my knowledge there is very, very little for lesbians who are HIV positive. Whether or not lesbians can get the virus through woman-to-woman sex, they do get it by other means, because lesbians can be injecting drug users, they may have been heterosexual in the not so distant past, or sleep with men from time to time now. What we are hoping to do in the health education group is develop a workshop which we can take to different groups of lesbians. In the first one we plan to target black women, and then perhaps next time we will modify it to target young women, or women who aren't identified as lesbians. We want to work in small groups so women feel safe to talk and are able to explore things in depth.

For me, one of the biggest issues for women about HIV prevention is in negotiating sex. This is a totally different thing for women than for men, and here I'm thinking more about heterosexual women than lesbians. Although negotiating safer sex is difficult for anyone, for heterosexual women it's also about women's more general role in society. A lot of information around about safer sex says: 'You get your partner to use a condom, okay?' That's it. But the reason women aren't practising safer sex more is because for a lot of us it's extremely difficult, it's not simple at all. Women have never found it particularly easy to get men to take birth-control seriously, and then, please, like suddenly they are going to be able to get men to agree to practise safer sex. And, of course it's supposed to be up to the woman to get men to do it! But in real life many things intervene in negotiating sex between men and women. Not the least is that women face real violence, or fear violence, from men. Also, a lot of women just aren't used to bringing up sex and talking about it.

Safer sex is especially hard for younger women to carry through. Younger women are not supposed to expect sex because if they do, they're slags. Sex always has to overcome you with passion. If you are prepared for the possibility of safer sex, you have to talk about it before it happens and then it's as if you are being a bit presumptuous. 'Oh, you think I want to sleep with you, oh really? Safer sex? Whoever said anything about sex?' There the young woman is laying herself on the line, and she runs the risk of being seen as 'easy' if she has condoms with her. You've got to wait for sex to happen, so how can you talk about it? I know from my own experience as a young woman that if you fancy someone, it's unlikely you're going to demand anything of them. If someone you really fancy actually likes you, it's wonderful; are you going to ask anything of them that might turn them off you? Like insist they wear a condom? Everything I'm describing is happening in a situation where the woman wants sex, but what about the many other young women who are pressured into having sex they don't really want? How do you deal with safer sex then? Not all young women are the same, but whoever they are, it seems that there are understandable reasons why practising safer sex is not simply the result of giving them 'correct' information. These are some of the difficulties young women (and many older ones too) face.

There is still an image around HIV that if you are a good, poor undeserving person, we're all going to feel sorry for you and see you as incredibly brave and strong if you're positive. But you have got to fulfil certain requirements to get sympathy: it helps to be well known, heterosexual, white, a man, and to have come from a respectable background. There is so much emphasis on how a person got the virus but at the end of the day, what difference does it make? You are a person, dealing with a possibly life-threatening condition, but the question of how you got it always remains. It's everywhere, in the press, even when doctors give reports they specify whether they are talking about heterosexual males or homosexuals. Why do they need to say it? It doesn't actually tell the person reading it anything apart from leading them to make an assessment of the positive person.

A man from the gutter press rang up Positively Women wanting to talk about a woman in Dallas, Texas, who was going around deliberately infecting people with HIV. I said we didn't have a response because it wasn't particularly relevant to our work. I couldn't prove or disprove that it happened but it certainly wasn't the main issue for women who are HIV positive. By printing the story the press was giving it a lot of energy and it would perpetuate the idea that the public (whoever they are) have good reason to fear people who are positive, which is not the case. It was disgusting. Then he asked me if we were finding that it was women from high risk groups like drug users who were still getting the virus, or was it more ordinary people? I had to tell him that there is no such thing as a high risk group, only high risk behaviour. He started to get stroppy with me because I wasn't playing, and yet it's not exactly news that it's behaviour, not identity, which is risky in relation to HIV.

A few years ago there was the green monkey rubbish which supposedly explained that HIV originated in Africa. Even now there are stories about HIV among heterosexuals being an imported disease. This is dangerous stuff in two ways: it gives other people a false sense of security, and it means that African people get a hard time whether they are positive or not. HIV is very frightening and some people want convenient scapegoats, easily identifiable ones, so that so-called ordinary people don't have to worry. If you keep identifying HIV as the problem of another group of people, gay or African, you can maintain your prejudices, hide your fear, and distance yourself. It is easier to be angry with somebody else than to come to terms with a virus than can affect anyone.

It's an aggravating and frustrating situation because there is good information around already. But the good material is not always being used or taken up, and people are still ignorant. There is 'official' HIV education coming from HIV organizations, but there is also the 'unofficial' HIV education coming from newspapers. This tells people that the figures are being exaggerated, that unless you are African or a drug user, heterosexuals don't have to worry. They are still telling people to avoid casual sex, as if that's the answer. Imagine this couple having unprotected sex and the little HIV virus is just about to be transmitted when it realizes they're in love and it's a serious relationship. So it says, 'Oops, sorry, my mistake'. Please.

Having said that, I also know that people can get conflicting messages even from good health education material. For instance, there are still confusions around the sexual guidelines and daily life guidelines to do with transmission of the virus. The Health Education Authority emphasizes that there is no danger from children who are HIV positive going to ordinary schools, which is absolutely correct. But on the other hand, in the sexual practice guidelines, there is a heavy emphasis on avoiding *any* exchange of blood or bodily fluid. If you are careless once, it could be you. People read about these two separate situations and are concerned about each one. Anybody knows that kids fall in the playground and scrape themselves, teachers are not always there, and kids may try to help the one who's hurt. If there is no danger from infected blood in that situation, why is there so much danger from infected blood or fluids in sex? People are not being silly when they wonder about these things and get confused. It's taken me a while to get a good sense of it. The reason why you have to be so careful in sex is that it's different from ordinary contact with blood; it involves bits of you inside your body and the blood or secretions go straight there. Whereas if a child cuts themselves, they might be bleeding but how is it going to get inside your body? It's difficult to get across because sometimes it's hard to be simple without losing the sense. It's not just bodily fluid or the blood in itself. It has to get into you and that doesn't happen at all easily in ordinary social situations. I don't blame the public for being confused because people can only draw conclusions from the information they get and they have had a lot of conflicting information. They take it and try to fit it into their lives. With sex, they want to believe they're safe because they don't really want to have to practise safer sex - the fear factor is often outweighed by their desire to continue having unsafe sex, or inability to negotiate safer sex. But the fear which the gutter press whips up towards people who are HIV positive outweighs the factual information and leads to a situation in which positive people, including children, can be rejected or feared.

I feel angry, frustrated, but not at all surprised at the level of racism surrounding HIV/AIDS. Researchers spending so much money trying to prove that AIDS came from Africa. It was first identified in America, but no, it has to come from Africa. Every theory that has come up so far has been discredited. Will they stop to look somewhere else?

I went to a lecture at St Thomas' hospital about HIV positive Africans living here and sexually transmitted diseases. The researcher had asked all these questions about the subjects' sexual histories, as well as how long they had been in this country. But he didn't ask them anything about their medical histories before they came to this country except to find out if they'd had a blood transfusion. If they hadn't had one, the assumption was made that they got the virus through heterosexual contact. But it could have happened through any number of other medical procedures, such as the use of unsterilized scalpels or needles. With statistics you only get answers to the questions you ask and in this case there were a lot of unasked questions.

Africa seems to be one big laboratory where researchers from Europe and America can go and study the effects of HIV or try out new drugs and then take the results home with them. I heard a doctor say that AZT is not appropriate for Africa because it's too expensive. When you put that together with the inferior services black people are getting here and in America, you realize that this is pretty deep, that our lives aren't worth so much, and that our deaths aren't so tragic.

I'm relatively new to the HIV field, but I don't feel as if I've just arrived because some of the issues are very familiar to me. When I first got into women's issues, I kept hearing that we were all women together and sexism was the issue. Racism was the little extra burden that black women (only) suffered from white men (only). It is similar with HIV, that is the big issue and we are all in this together. Well, the differences between us are very important and if there is not a clear awareness of them, sexism gets defined in terms of how it affects white middle-class women and HIV gets defined in terms of how it affects white men. With racism tacked on as an optional extra. I have heard of black women being tested for HIV in ante-natal clinics without their consent, now. Black people are being refused entry to Britain because the might be HIV positive and because they haven't got enough money to pay for treatment they might need if they got ill. That sort of stuff isn't a side issue. It has to be central to any discussion of 'HIV issues'. It is all right to talk about racism out there: the National Front, South Africa, so we can all say 'Oh, how terrible.' But to raise things here and now about the racism that black women are having as users and workers in HIV organizations is very different and you can suddenly become Miss Unpopular. For a lot of black women racism is like an invisible page added to your job description.

At Positively Women I am responsible for the training of and working with the voluntary and statutory sector. At the moment I'm trying to squeeze that into something more manageable because the voluntary and statutory sector is everybody. I see myself developing more of a focus for our own courses, doing things around women's issues, and working with the people who do training around these issues. Very importantly, I'm going to be putting on more training workshops for clients. To my mind there is a lot of energy put into training for people who aren't HIV positive or who are untested, but when you are HIV positive there isn't that much on offer. For instance, assertiveness is an important issue for positive women. It may sound vague and woolly but in this context it's quite specific: it's about feeling strong in yourself and able to keep your head together, being able to be demanding. Some doctors can be good, but some can be rude or dismissive; positive women will probably see doctors more regularly than other women and it's important that they're able to feel more in control. Assertiveness is necessary in order to have some control in your life and involvement in what is happening to you.

We also get lots of requests to send someone to give a talk on women and HIV. There are more positive women around who could do it but who might want to gain the necessary skills to take on that task with confidence. More positive women might like to do training for telephone and other forms of counselling; that would be good for Positively Women and for the women themselves because they could build on their own experiences and develop important skills, as well as helping other women in the same situation. More women could be trained to know what positive people's rights are, so they could give advice to other women who contact us. The educational side of my work includes developing materials and leaflets. At the moment I'm working on an African women's leaflet as well as revamping our existing ones. All in all my job is a bit untidy but a job in any voluntary organization is that way - large and untidy.

We are more and more aware at Positively Women of the fact that the organization is changing; this is not simply a matter of having taken on more staff. We don't only run support groups any more, we tackle other areas and have different specialties; my position is in training and education, another is in development, and a third is as a children's worker, and these are only the new positions. Once we acknowledge that the organization is changing, it's fine. I am taking a course now about managing in the voluntary and non-profit sector and we are looking at what happens when there is change, how tensions can be caused, especially when the organization started off as a small self-help group made up of a few people who get to know each other really well. At that stage it's relatively easy to decide what you want to do and how to do it. At Positively Women we now have ten employed women and we are all running in and out of the office all the time, so sometimes I don't see one of my co-workers for a week at a time. We've had to become much more structured. This is an issue for me because I've not been here long and I can see quite clearly that women who have been here longer were much more used to a looser and more spontaneous form of working. At the moment everyone is putting a fair amount of energy into being an organization and developing different types of structures. When we've accomplished the initial phases of that, we'll have more time to develop in other ways; right now it's necessary to establish who we are, what we do, and what our priorities are.

It's necessary and good that Positively Women is changing. We're going to start developing more groups for specific groups of women where we look at particular groups, see what their needs are, and then organize to meet those needs. We are also focusing more on the training and development side of things. Time will tell how we handle the changes. We are going to have to find our niche rather than trying to do everything. We are, even in our expanded state, a tiny organization, the organization for positive women. People want us to give more than we can because there aren't any other specific women's organizations. But we need to consolidate and to be clear about who we are. If we could develop regionally that would be wonderful but it's not going to happen in a hurry.

For every woman who finds Positively Women, there are many others who don't. The numbers of people who are going to be living with HIV is getting bigger and bigger, and those people are going to have needs; yet there are indications that the money available to AIDS organizations is not going to increase. It's clear from research in the United States that if you are positive, the quality of your life makes a huge difference to the amount of time you survive. These differences are most starkly seen between comfortably-off gay men and very poor black women in New York City; it's a difference which can be measured in the number of years you survive with HIV. We know how important provisions and equal rights are to women who are HIV positive. We try to meet those needs today; tomorrow we will have an even bigger job.

FACING THE
CHALLENGE -
LIVING WITH 'IT'!

ANDRIA EFTHIMIOU

*Andria is a thirty-one-year-old woman of
Greek Cypriot ethnic origin. Her
involvement with HIV began in 1987
when one of her closest friends was
diagnosed HIV positive. In her own
words she 'read every HIV-related book,
article or leaflet I could get my hands on'
in order to equip herself emotionally and
with information. Since 1988, she has
worked with HIV positive drug users, as
an advocacy worker and counsellor. In
1988 she met John who has AIDS and has
been with him ever since.*

WHEN I FIRST started to write, I was feeling very confident
and together, as though anything were possible. Today I don't
feel that as much. I always present a very 'bravado' image,
but when it comes down to really letting go and spilling the
beans, it isn't so easy. Well, it isn't. AIDS raises so many
anxieties and questions for people. Writing about it in such
an uncertain atmosphere while trying to be positive, takes real
effort. These are very intimate issues.

How I met John was quite strange in itself. I was studying

at polytechnic and had set up an AIDS Awareness Group where students and staff could come to discuss and get information and support around any HIV/AIDS related issues. To be honest, I didn't really know what I was doing. As an ex-injecting drug user, some of whose friends had been diagnosed HIV positive, I just felt I had to do something. Also listening to my fellow students around the lunch-time tables, preening their feathers and mouthing off about all their unsafe sexual conquests was frightening.

Anyway, I thought I'd better find out a bit more and get some direction from people who were used to doing this kind of work consistently. I visited the Terrence Higgins Trust and they immediately referred me to Frontliners. Who? I had never even heard of them at the time. They had offices just above the Trust, so I went straight up. I quickly learned that Frontliners is a self-help group/organization for people with ARC or AIDS, run by people with ARC or AIDS.

I was introduced to a man named John F who was skinny and gay and very kind; before long we had a great rapport with each other. When he heard that the college AIDS Awareness Group had been organizing benefits and raising money, he was quick to point out that Frontliners' money goes directly to people living with HIV, and therefore I should give whatever we raised straight to him! There's nothing like an assertive queen!

After about thirty minutes of chatting, I felt really comfortable. I'm not exactly a shy retiring type myself, so I told him I was an ex-injecting drug user, after which he almost immediately suggested I meet Frontliners' Drug Liaison Officer, another man named John M. I responded in no uncertain terms that I didn't need to see him as I no longer used drugs. Also, I wasn't a woman living with ARC or AIDS. No, no, he said, he just meant that he thought I shared a lot of similar ideas and thoughts with this man, and that there weren't that many people around who were as concerned about drug users and HIV as he and I obviously were. (I'd already been kicked out of working in a therapeutic community as a result of opening my mouth at a conference to say things, which today people get applauded for - but we can't all be trendsetters like me!)

I agreed to meet John, Frontliners' Drug Liaison Officer, during the following week. When I arrived, I remember being led into one of the small rooms next door to Frontliners by John F who reminded me cheekily not to get up to 'anything' as he'd be listening at the keyhole. Nothing was further from my mind.

So I met John M and we talked a lot about ourselves - the usual anger, pain and joy of any two recovering addicts. It was a very safe meeting and before I knew it we were sharing quite intimate details of our lives, one of which was that he was maintained on a methadone script. If I'd been interested in him in any other way, that information soon withered the thoughts out of my mind. I told him I wanted to get rid of the first bit of money our Poly group had raised through a sponsored dance and he, of course, was only too willing to take it, at which point the meeting more or less ended. Except that I asked him if he and another Frontliner would come and speak at an AIDS Awareness Day I had organized at my college. He agreed.

On the day, I met John in the student's cafeteria where we chatted for a few minutes. I was surprised that he was early; I'm always late for everything and the only reason I was early that day was because I was the organizing the event! Half way through the day I had a phone call from a male friend who is in my ex-users' self-help group to say that he really did want to run the safer sex workshop, so we arranged an impromptu cab for him and much was learnt by all.

After this successful event, we all travelled home together and I ended up asking John if he wanted to come to my house for supper one day. We made the arrangement, and he carried on talking to my other friend as if nothing had happened! By this stage I had started wondering what was going on inside of me, but I tried not to think about it too much.

There are a few thing you need to know now in order to understand the events I'm about to relate to you. After I left rehab, I decided I wouldn't have anyone round to my home who was still using anything apart from alcohol, and that was only because most people drink and it was too insane to block them out too! This decision, which I had been sticking to, meant that I had a problem on my hands about my invitation to John and I was in a bit of an emotional dilemma. I quickly phoned him up, told him why, and said I'd come round to his place instead. He was a bit taken aback but took it in his stride. (Since then, I have come to be more inclusive of people in my social circles, as I have come to terms with my own past and my own addiction.)

Anyway, I went round expecting a meal, and we ended up at the Indian take-away. We ate, and talked for ages and ages. I really liked him and I guess inside I had already decided to stay with him - but I kept thinking I was completely insane. I mean, he could die next week. Yes, the other side of my head would say, but then again there's always today. And then I started imagining that I had all sorts of other ulterior motives. Looking back, these seem to have amounted to nothing. The fact is, this person was just right for me. He was bold, he didn't really care what other people thought, he did what he felt was right. He was warm and strong, all in all a warm and coura- geous individual who I strongly identified with. He also had ten times more self-esteem than me. His particular hell had been much more intense than mine, particularly his experience of being deported from China as a result of being HIV posi- tive. So we started a relationship that night.

It wasn't easy for me. I had to go 'in the closet' in my own support group because I knew I would be condemned for hav- ing a relationship with a 'using addict'. After three months of this, I told John that I couldn't do it anymore. I even convinced myself I was in love with someone else - for four hellish days.

Actually most of our relationship has been nothing but posi- tive for both of us. The first night we were together, I picked up a bottle of tablets from the table and asked what they were. He answered that they were anti-depressants given to him af- ter a suicide attempt. When I asked if he still used them, he said no. I was just about to throw them in the bin when I remembered one of the strong messages of my self-help group, which is to stop trying to 'control' people, places and things. I left them on the table and the next time we met they'd been thrown away by John himself. Sometimes a gentle reminder is all it takes. John also withdrew himself from chlorpromazine, an anti-psychotic drug. God knows what he was doing on it in the first place; he's not psychotic as far as I know!

Then I had to work through whether his bottle of methadone was going to suddenly sprout legs and jump down my throat. Apparently not - I had a choice in the matter. John had to have it for pain control in any case.

During all this time I was doing my finals at college and getting into the studying. The AIDS work had to go on, and as well, there was a student occupation of the college. John kept calling me a radical and telling me to get on with my studying, but I had to support the 'action'. Also a good friend of mine had finally decided to come off drugs and she was really ill in hospital, so I was visiting her as much as possible. I started walking into walls but as far as I was concerned all of this had to go on.

Anyway, sex! I'm waffling on trying to avoid the trickier subjects. When I first sat down to write, I felt I had to put down the intricate details of our sexual behaviour, but since then I've had second thoughts, and I know John wouldn't like it either. There are a few things that are significant though. One is that people are always asking me if I'm scared of becoming HIV positive. And I have to say that in the beginning I was a lot more scared than I am now. In a nutshell, that says it all. I have been tested since we've been together and I have remained negative. Even though we follow the safer sex guidelines, there are niggling fears from time to time. However, generally I'm not afraid.

Safer sex is okay. It's good fun actually. What bothers me more is that I can't have a child which is John's. Or I could, but it would mean living in fear while we waited to see whether the baby or I became positive. I don't want to have to cope with that. I keep thinking I may change my mind, but right now I don't think either of us could live with it. Basically, the way we see it is that if we took the risk and I had a baby, what if we were both diagnosed positive? It is possible I would then be left with a painful legacy from John which isn't what either of us want. If he did die before me, I would rather remember all the crazy and exciting things we've done together and how happy we were, doing things like trying to visit the whole globe and experience 'everything' rapido! God, it's been manic sometimes. This includes an internal sense of urgency which is both overwhelmingly sad (because it is the constant reminder of why we should need to do so much so quickly), and exhausting. Sometimes I find myself symbolically and actually on my knees praying and wishing that someone would come, wave a hand and make it all better again.

As far as being a woman affected by AIDS goes, I'm often angry or in pain about the fact that I can't be myself in many situations. Consequently, I sometimes find myself declaring the fact that my partner has AIDS in the most inappropriate situations just because I'm so furious. Of course those women who are supportive have been very supportive, but those who haven't have been so hard at times. What really infuriates me is the fact that I live in a world where people are segregated and discriminated against because they're gay, black, working class, or whatever. But prejudice and harassment (which we have both had) when you're ill is totally sick. I understand about the rationales: fear and panic about AIDS, but that is no excuse; ultimately other peoples' fears about HIV are not our responsibility. Finally we all have to look at what we have, face it and get on and deal with each day as it comes.

For eighteen months John has maintained a good, long healthy streak. He feels he does the best he can to maintain his health and on the whole I agree. But there have been some very scary times too. One time recently, when I was stressed out from work, John's routine hospital check on the level of his blood coagulation showed that it wasn't coagulating at all. The doctors admitted him to hospital immediately and within six hours he'd haemorrhaged in his leg. It was quite terrifying, especially coupled with the fact that he'd had an unidentified chest infection for some time. I cried for five days; I thought the exhausting weeping was never going to stop. By the end of the week I really couldn't do much more than sleep and visit him in hospital. At times like these, my feelings have been so extreme; you can really exist in a ravine of despair where it's almost impossible to be reached by other human beings. I could be with one of John's health care workers or a friend, they might be trying to console me, but I would be gazing straight ahead, not really connecting at all. Ultimately that amount of pain is only yours, but the fact that someone extends a strong arm or a warm hand could mean acknowledging to yourself that you will not drown and die in it.

It's difficult to go for support when you're in a supportive role all day, but I guess it simply comes down to being unable to let go of your pride, and in my case, fear. I realize now that I don't trust people with my feelings, not because I feel they will stamp all over them, but because being vulnerable in itself is painful. With another person, it can be horrid! (It can also be wonderful!) But eventually I was forced to let go of all that and look for help. Besides, if I hadn't, I would have continued to dump everything on John which was making me feel guilty.

On the issue of drugs, the fact is that few people in my own support network could live with and accept my present circumstances. The ones who can seem to be people who are in the same situation themselves, or people who have not 'used' drugs for a very long time, or people who love and care about me anyway. Whatever, I have been alienated from a group which for a long time was my mainstay. I just wish people would stop projecting their fears on me. I appreciate concern but not obsessive fear and a little ignorance. The reality is that I have coped and no, it isn't easy sometimes, but I wonder how those who judge would have dealt with it all? It's only a few who actually say anything; it's the silence which is much more threatening and disturbing.

This has meant having to look elsewhere for support. I have been involved with a 'partners of people with AIDS' group which for most of the time has been all gay men and me - surprise, surprise! There are two men and me who have been involved in the group since the very beginning, we have become close and I have appreciated them greatly. For a while I was involved with ACT UP (AIDS Coalition to Unleash Power - an activist group), which gave me a place to channel my anger, but because of various issues, I found myself getting even more angry and decided to give it up for the time being.

Nothing has ever made me feel as strongly over such a long period of time as AIDS and what it is doing to the group of people who came to be my (first) extended family. That in itself is crucially important for me because I often get bored and give up after a short space of time. I have learned so much. People refer to both of us for information about things concerning HIV/AIDS and drug use, both nationally and internationally. It's good to feel that you're life is making a bit of difference to someone else's on the earth. It also stops you thinking about yourself all the time which, if you've been through as much therapy as I have (for addiction etc), is always a blessing.

Probably one of the most special and important things I want to say is that I have found a whole other group of people, some of whom are addicts and some of whom are not, who are respectful and inspiring in their determination to make the world a safer place for people with AIDS, and who will do almost anything to enable that to happen. I can relate to that! Meanwhile, getting on with the daily living and loving is what I intend to do. Loving is something we're pretty good at.

SEX IN
DIFFICULT TIMES

SUE O'SULLIVAN

*Sue O'Sullivan is one of the editors of
this book. She has a health education
background and worked in publishing for
many years.*

'IT ISN'T WHAT you do, it's the way that you do it.'
'If sex is so simple, how come we worry about it all the time?'
'Safer sex, huh! I had problems getting my boyfriend to take
birth-control seriously, and his attitude about HIV doesn't seem
very different.'

This is a chapter about women and sex. It isn't only about safer
sex. How can we deal with safer sex when there is so much
confusion, fear of rejection and lack of confidence about sex
in general? All this without even taking the virus into account;
and when we do take the virus into account, phew! There's
stigma and secrecy and fear of death. We have to begin to open
up and to contemplate the many layers of influences which affect
how we feel sexually, how we see ourselves in the world sexually (where ever we happen to be in it), how we do and don't
manage to acknowledge and negotiate the kinds of sexual relationships we want, and how we can begin to sort out our
positions as women in a world which is still largely male-
dominated.

Listen, we fall in love, we have sexual desires, we want sexual
satisfaction, and we want to please our lovers. Many of us want

to be with men, some of us want women, and others fancy both sexes. Many of us have discovered the delights of pleasuring ourselves through masturbation. But in different ways, within different contexts, most of us at some point in our lives are caught up in sexual attractions or pressures and the reality of having sex with someone else. If someone is ill or feeling sick, sex may be the last thing on their mind, but they may regret the loss of that possibility, even if it is only temporary. There are times as well, when we may have no desire for sex of any kind. This is fine. Many women have discovered that in celibacy they found peace and relief at being out of the domain of sexual tension and expectation. Their lives have been as rich and varied as anyone else's.

It's only if sex is regarded as a variety of sexual acts that we can approach the subject in a relatively straightforward way. Even if that were possible, difficulties remain. After all, what is sex? What is 'real' sex? When sex between a man and a woman is being described, as in 'they had sex', whose sexual pleasure is being described? Is it the man's orgasm, achieved through intercourse, which defines having sex? What about kissing and stroking? Clitoral stimulation? Penetration with fingers? Oral sex? Is it 'real' sex if the woman doesn't have an orgasm? Is it 'real' sex if the woman or the man has an orgasm through any other means except penetration? Do orgasms matter? Does penetration matter to all women? Do two women making love have 'real' sex? It's time that women finally changed the definitions of sex altogether - 'real' sex is what brings mutual pleasure, full stop.

Some of us may know what we like, or wish we could try out or discover in practice. If we are heterosexual, penetration may not be our main aim. Even then, we may still believe that fucking is the only 'real' sex. For so long everything else has been described as foreplay that even if we're the lucky recipients of it and know that it can be, or is, the most pleasurable aspect of sex (and perhaps the only way we can get orgasms), somehow we feel it isn't as good as penetration. Of course none of this means that many women don't love penetration, love fucking. Of course they do, but that doesn't invalidate the equally large number of women who don't, or the even larger numbers who value a whole variety of sexual acts equally, or who like one thing one time, and another the next time. Lots of women know this is a ridiculous state of affairs but because heterosexual women's sexual desires are obviously intertwined with men, and because so many men are trapped in a mind and body set which only really values fucking, we go along with it.

Why do women go along with it? At the risk of sounding like an old record, a lot of it is because men still call the tune. Women may have come a long way in discarding feelings of inadequacy and second-rate status in relation to men, but many still feel vulnerable and lack confidence in sexual matters. This pattern of thought isn't only an attitude, it accurately reflects the power and prestige men still hold relative to women in our society.

But we don't have to be defined as victims of forces outside ourselves. Even if it's difficult, even if we have mixed feelings, women can make changes in their lives, including their sexual lives. Let's set the record straight. Sex, between anybody, may include penetration, whether it's with a penis, fingers, a dildo, or a nice fresh (and washed) cucumber. Penetration itself has many different moods, from sweaty lust, to deliberate, skilled thrusts. But sex is also touching, soft with gentle fingers, firm and holding, hard and pushing, squeezing. It's kissing, sweet, long, probing, feathery, wet, demanding and hungry. It's using lips and tongue on the body, tracing paths on backs, inside thighs, across an instep, on nipples. It's blowing breath on genitals, brushing clits, sucking and stroking with mouth and tongue, pushing fingers into cunts, holding pricks in mouths, tickling balls with fingernails. Sex is teasing around arseholes, it's sucking nipples and pressing and kissing and lying on top, and rolling around, and using sex toys like vibrators.

Sex is getting turned on - before, during, again. It may include having orgasms - sometimes, often, rarely. It's hundreds of variations, or only a few. It's passionate and intense, hilarious, boring, disastrous, satisfying, clumsy, expert, wanted, ordinary. It's simple, tried and true, or complicated and brand new. It's experimental, it's comfortable, it's scary, it's with a new partner, or an old love. It happens when you're young, middle-aged, old. It happens between men and women, women and women, men and men, and let's not forget, on your own. It has different meanings in different cultures. It has different boundaries and rules attached to it in different cultures and different historical times. It is not separate from the rest of our lives or concerns. We see it around us constantly, we read about it, we talk about it. And yet it remains, for the most part, an act between two people, carried out in private.

Yes, we talk about sex: with our closest friends, maybe to our doctor. But not very often with our partner. When we're girls and the talking could really help exploration, or the use of birth-control, or the drawing of boundaries, or the use of safer sex, it's difficult. Boys still seem to think that the girl who talks about sex before it happen, expects it to happen. Therefore she's a slut. They think, if she's prepared and carrying a condom, then she must plan to have sex - with me! Clearly we need to change a lot more than helping girls feel more confident about negotiating safer sex!

What this illustrates is that even if we're grown-up women, sex doesn't happen in a vacuum. We are people who live in the world, who have histories, aspirations and dreams, and who experience contradictions in our lives. And so do our partners. Our desires do not spring, ready made, from our genitals. They are complicated things, not reducible to so-called 'natural' drives.

Which brings us to safer sex. We all know about the 'rules' of safer sex. They are on one level very simple. No exchange of bodily fluids or blood in which the HIV virus may be present. In sexual terms this is most important when considering semen. The ground rule of safer sex is no semen in the vagina or anus. Everything else is more or less open to interpretation or individual decisions. Of course the virus is present in other bodily fluids, including vaginal fluids, but the highest concentration is in semen and blood. But wait a minute: what about everything we've been talking about - the difficulties of reducing sex to straightforward physical acts, the problems of teasing sex out from other layers of influence and constraint? The complexity of relationships, especially with men? Is it true that everyone, HIV positive or not, should be practising safer sex? If sex is more than fucking, if 'real' sex is a variety of sexual activities, what about those activities? And what about the possibility of transmission of the virus from vaginal fluids?

All of us, to a greater of lesser degree, have problems about safer sex, and that includes positive women. Those women who are not positive, or do not know their status, may think of safer sex in terms of remaining free of the virus, but in our sexual relationships we are all subject to fears of rejection, fears of labelling or stigmatizing, and desires for intimacy and pleasure. If heterosexual, we have to negotiate our sexual relationships through sexism, and assumptions about women, whether we are positive or not, and this isn't always easy. It's important to realize too, that even if a man is the most tender, understanding person in the world, and sees his female partner as equal, the pervasiveness of sexual inequality is such that the woman may still fear rejection or difficulty if she insists on safer sex.

I've been concentrating on the complexity of sex so much because it's been far too simplified in so much safer sex material. When it turns out not to be such a simple task, we may feel that we've failed. We may give up, or give up sex, or feel guilty and bad if we haven't managed it 100 per cent of the time. What is needed is some understanding and acceptance of the complexity of the different situations we find ourselves in, and the knowledge that if we fail from time to time, we are not bad, and we can help ourselves to make safer choices the next time. This is true, no matter what our HIV status is.

Of course it is particularly important that positive women explore their own situations, perhaps with other positive women and with their partners. Positive women do not turn into saints the minute they know they are positive. Why should anyone expect that? But positive women are living with HIV, and therefore, by that very fact, living with the reality in all aspects of their lives. Positive women may have heightened fears of rejection by their partners, and their partners may be ambiguous about not wanting to reject their positive lover. That may become symbolized by a refusal to wear a condom. They may even have a romantic urge to share the risks with her. Positive women also have to take on board the knowledge that to become re-infected with the HIV virus could worsen their health. The question of pregnancy is also important to some positive women. A climate which assumes that positive women should not have a baby, even though the risk of passing the virus to the baby is lower than originally thought, means that those women who desperately want one have few recourses other than unprotected sex with a man.

Too often the assumption made by heterosexuals who are not positive, or do not know their status, is that all will be fine if they avoid having sex with positive people. This is off beam in a number of ways. In the first place there are positive people who do not know their status. Positive people are ordinary people; it's ridiculous to think you can tell that someone is positive by looking at them. In the second place what does this say about positive people? That they are unworthy of being fancied? Or loved? Of course they are worthy of both. Also HIV is a weak virus. It is a dangerous virus when it finds a home, but it can be quite easily shut out by, yes, practising safer sex, and not sharing injecting equipment when using drugs intravenously. By practising the ground rules of safer sex, no semen in the vagina or anus, which obviously means that the man should use an approved variety of condom every time he penetrates a woman vaginally or anally, the risks of transmission of the virus from a man to a woman, or a woman to a man, will be hugely reduced.

As far as deciding whether or not you need to use safer sex, it is absolutely important to be 100 per cent certain that you can and do communicate honestly and clearly with your lover, and that it is reciprocated. Can you talk honestly and openly about your sexual and drug-related histories covering the past ten years or more? Do you believe your partner can? These are difficult questions to weigh up and it seems reasonable to at least take on safer sex as an important necessity in any new relationship. How often do people know each other inside out before they have sex together? How often do established relationships harbour sexual secrets, or hidden pasts? Taking on these complexities is an essential part of making decisions about safer sex, whoever you are.

There are disagreements about what constitutes the practice of safer sex and all the other sexual activities which people can and do explore. Information is contradictory, opinions range far and wide, new knowledge brings new guidelines and advice. And emotions are not always in tune with knowledge - sometimes a positive person may be scared of kissing, even though she knows it is not a risky activity, because she's frightened of passing the virus on, and thinks, 'What if...'. The lover who is not positive may harbour fears of kissing, with similar knowledge of its lack of danger, because of a persistent voice saying, 'What if they're wrong and it can happen this way?' These feelings are understandable but they can change. Our feelings don't remain static and if they're not shoved under the carpet, ease can replace unease.

What are the current guidelines on safer sex and non-penetrative sexual activities? Again we have to understand that nothing is fully understood and different 'experts' give different advice. We may desperately want total answers but they don't always exist. Learning to live with an element of uncertainty about HIV transmission is part of living in the time of AIDS, but uncertainty is not a new phenomenon. We live with uncertainty about other aspects of our lives. For up-to-date guidelines we have to get current advice and remember that because HIV and AIDS are not understood in any complete way, we have to look to new information as it is available and then try to build our own framework in which to fit the advice. This is the difficult part. No one can tell us for sure exactly what is and isn't safe apart from unprotected fucking in the vagina or anus.

Oral sex is a case in point. Lots of women adore getting oral sex. Is it risky? Advice directed at heterosexual women sometimes doesn't even mention it, and when it does, rarely in detail. Some advice indicates that it is a very low risk sexual practice. However, some lesbians and heterosexual women feel strongly that oral sex is a real and present risk, although not as risky as unprotected penile penetration, and that it is possible to transmit the virus through licking and sucking a woman's clitoris and vaginal area. Other women believe oral sex is so close to being totally safe that no one should be frightened of it. Most suggest that you should abstain from oral sex if the woman being licked has her period. One of the problems in evaluating women's risks from HIV is that the research, classifications, and surveys done to present have not concentrated on transmission from women to men or to women. There is anecdotal evidence that a few people have been infected from practising oral sex alone, usually when the woman has had her period. Wider anecdotal evidence suggests that it is not a risky activity. In other words very few people are reported to have acquired the virus through oral sex. In the decade or more that we have been aware of the virus, thousands of positive people have engaged in oral sex with partners who are not positive and who have not become infected.

But that doesn't mean you might not be worried about it, or that anyone can say that no one at all has, or won't become infected through oral sex. Right now the way to deal with that worry or uncertainty is either to stop doing oral sex, or to work through the worry and decide that in your evaluation of the risk, it's okay to go ahead, or to use a barrier and lick through it. It also seems sensible to advise everyone to play it safer and avoid going down on a woman while she has her period, or to always use a barrier then. Dental dams were invented for use in dental surgery but have been co-opted by oral safer sex fans. These are latex squares which are held over the vaginal area by either partner. This isn't always easy to get the hang of, so some people have invented crotchless knickers with latex sewn in so the licking partner has his or her hands free. Dental dams aren't easy to come by (see RESOURCES at the end of the book); an alternative is to cut the tip off a condom and then cut it length wise - the advice is to use a water based lubricant on the clit and vagina and then hold the latex over it. Licking lube off of latex isn't very tasty. The use of cling film as a barrier to HIV is doubtful, but it might be the material you use the first time in order to get the 'feel' of doing it.

As far as sucking off a man goes, the advice is again contradictory. In Britain the emphasis is on safer sex for fucking; currently the Terrence Higgins Trust does not advise men that blow jobs are risky. But others disagree. Similar anecdotal evidence exists about men being infected by having oral sex with other men as exists about cunnilingus (licking and sucking a woman's clitoris and vagina). However, if there is any worry or unease, the man can wear a condom. Some women love sucking their partner's prick, but others are put off, perhaps by the idea of semen in their mouth. In this case, a condom might be attractive to a woman and give her partner a pleasure he hadn't had with her before.

Latex gloves are the accompaniment for other forms of sex in which one or both of the partners are worried that the activity may be risky. Again there is little or no evidence that anyone has become positive through putting their fingers in a vagina, or even an arsehole, let alone in a mouth. We have all heard about cuts and sores allowing the virus in, or transmitting the virus to the body it is in. But remember, those cuts and sores would have to be open and bleeding in order for even theoretical transmission to take place. Latex gloves enable a worried man or woman to finger fuck. They can also be used when you want to stimulate the anus. Lube can be used for vaginal finger fucking with gloves, but you must always use it if you are going to penetrate the anus. Always check safer sex guidelines to see which kinds of lubes to use with latex. Latex gloves can be found in certain chemists and from some sex shops, particularly gay ones. (See RESOURCES.)

Sex toys are safer sex friendly. These include things like vibrators and dildos as well as silk scarves, lotions, body oils, and sexy stories, among hundreds of other things. Fucking with a dildo is safe. The only proviso is that you wash it carefully with soap and water between shares. You can use a condom on sex toys like vibrators and dildos but remember, change it before you share the toy. A dildo is not a penis. The whole point is that you can have penetration if you want, finish, wash it up and toss it in your drawer. Not the same as a penis at all.

Remember that nothing that is being described here is necessary for you to do. For instance, some women may be shocked and horrified by the idea of a dildo, or of oral sex. There is no reason to disguise that. Sit down and think about it for a while. Where does the shock or disgust come from? Maybe it's only because it's something unknown. Maybe it's because it goes against everything you were ever taught or believed. Perhaps you have a history of sexual abuse. Whatever your answer, knowing about something doesn't mean you have to try it out or even if you do try it, like it, or ever do it again. One thing which HIV and AIDS has taught us is that we have to admit to the realms of possibility everything sexual which is consensual and practised by human beings. How else can we talk about sex and stopping the transmission of HIV and include everyone in the discussion?

Safer sex is primarily about HIV transmission. But it also has relevance for wider health concerns. Positive women will want to conserve their health; common sexually transmitted diseases (STDs) may have more serious negative effects on an HIV positive woman. No one wants to get hepatitis, gonorrhoea, thrush, or herpes, but for a positive woman it is even more important to avoid these, and safer sex can protect from a lot more than HIV. There is also evidence which suggests that the presence of an STD heightens the possibility of HIV transmission. When considering STDs, the use of latex squares for oral sex can be important.

Sex is a complicated business. It's not everything in life, but it can be puzzling and compelling. Let's take it seriously but not be too hard on ourselves or others. Success or failure isn't the best way to look at anything which is in process. Learning how to negotiate sex is difficult and ongoing, and includes trying and failing, trying and getting part way there, and trying successfully. For positive women the pressure may be intensified and the desire to get to grips with it greater. One of the biggest blocks we all have around sex is that we believe we're the only ones who have ambivalences or problems in sexual matters and so we stumble on feeling as if we're at fault. But we all have them, whether we're positive or not, and they definitely don't go away with a positive diagnosis. Opening up and talking about sex with a partner, a friend, within a group of friends, often dispels this myth. Sharing our ambivalences, our contradictory feelings, and our desires to be a responsible person about HIV and AIDS helps us to demystify the process and make it more possible to play an active, confident part in our sexual relationships, whoever we are.

HEALTH
INFORMATION
&
RESOURCES

MEDICAL TREATMENT IN HIV DISEASE

DR DAVID O'FLYNN

*David O'Flynn was born in London
in 1960. He qualified as a doctor
and as a psychiatrist, and is currently
working as a research psychiatrist
at Guy's Hospital in London.*

A NUMBER OF interventions by doctors are now possible in HIV infection and disease. There are some general points to consider before looking at the strategies used by doctors and the effects and side-effects of the drugs themselves.

The medical model demands that drugs are proved to be effective and relatively safe rather than just seeming to be so. Proof is usually established in clinical trials. In the simplest trial a group of patients is split into two - one half is given the treatment under investigation; the other half is given a placebo or another proven treatment. The progress of the disease is then compared in the two groups. Any difference is attributed to the treatment. This process is then repeated in a number of different groups as if only one trial is done, a difference may due to chance.

Clinical trials are time consuming. This process of testing drugs in HIV disease and the resulting delay in delivering drugs to all people has been criticized. The results of these trials are rarely straightforward. Often trials have statistical or design problems that shed doubt on their results. The majority of trials in HIV disease have been done on groups of men. For these reasons it is important if you are recommended a treatment that you ask doctors, nurses, health advisors and voluntary sector agencies for information on the effectiveness of the drugs and on their safety. As the treatment of HIV disease is progressing the information and advice here will change. Ultimately, decisions about treatment are yours.

There are four conventional medical strategies:

1 **DIRECT ACTION ON HIV - ANTI-HIV ANTI-VIRAL DRUGS**
   These drugs slow the replication, the production of HIV therefore slowing the damage to the immune system. A number of studies have demonstrated the effectiveness of this approach. There is controversy about their use but doctors agree on their value. With these drugs there tends to be some recovery in the immune system as well.

2 **TREATMENT OF DISEASES ARISING FROM IMMUNE DEFICIENCY - OPPORTUNISTIC INFECTIONS AND MALIGNANCIES**
   There are over one hundred opportunistic conditions associated with HIV disease - information will be limited to the common ones.

3 **PROPHYLAXIS AGAINST OPPORTUNISTIC INFECTIONS**
   This is the regular use of a drug in the absence of disease to prevent the disease. It has been suggested that half the improvement in the health of those with HIV disease has been due to anti-HIV anti-viral drugs and half due to prophylaxis against pneumocystis carinii, an organism causing pneumonia (PCP). Prophylaxis tends to use drugs used in the treatment of the disease (See point 2) but in lower doses.

4 STIMULATION OF THE IMMUNE SYSTEM

While there are no established methods to do this there may be in the near future. Reports (1991) on the use of vaccines in people with HIV disease show promise, but this work is at an early stage. The only drug that has been on trial - Immuthiol - has recently been withdrawn as people receiving it were doing worse than those in the matched (control) group.

ANTI-HIV ANTI-VIRAL DRUGS

AZT (Azidothymidine, Zidovudine Retrovir)

AZT is the only licensed drug for use as an anti-HIV anti-viral. AZT has been established as helpful in early and late HIV disease. Trials also suggest it is helpful for people with asymptomatic HIV infection when there is evidence of decline in immunity. The principal test used is the CD4 cell (T-cell) count - a measure of the number of a particular cell in the blood. Treatment with AZT is recommended if the CD4 cell count is below 500. People without HIV infection might be expected to have CD4 counts of around 1000. Symptoms can be expected as the numbers fall, and generally below 100 people have severely impaired immunity, and will have opportunistic disease. It is important to remember:

a) many people with very low CD4 counts (i.e. under fifty) have little or no disease
b) CD4 counts are very variable in one person
c) a trend over several months probably gives a clearer picture than one measure
d) people should judge their health principally by how they feel, and which symptoms they have, rather than by last month's CD4 count. The decision to accept AZT - i.e. daily medication for the foreseeable future - when asymptomatic, raises issues for many people.

The dose varies from 400mg to 1g or more a day. Originally AZT was taken at four to six hourly intervals with an emphasis on regular and punctual administration. (Hence the chorus of timer bleeps at a gathering of people on it.) It is now thought these restrictions and high doses are not necessary and most people will be offered 250mg twice daily. AZT is taken as a tablet.

SIDE-EFFECTS

i) Anaemia

This is a direct effect of the drug on the bone marrow. Other types of blood cell can also be suppressed. Anaemia is a common reason for dose reductions or withdrawal of the treatment. The anaemia may require transfusion. Anaemia seems more common in people with either low CD4 counts (less than 100) or advanced disease. Chronic use of paracetamol has been suggested to increase the chance of these problems - but the evidence changes regularly.

ii) Nausea, headache, rash, abdominal pain, fever, muscle pains, pins and needles, insomnia, anorexia, malaise, dizziness, sweating, shortness of breathe, heartburn, anxiety, loss of mental acuity, depression, chills, coughs and a flu-like syndrome. These are listed more or less in order of frequency. These are much less common now lower doses of drug are being used. Many of course could be related to the disease rather than the treatment.

iii) Pregnancy and lactation - there is no information. The risks of the drug in pregnancy are unknown. Breast-feeding is not recommended.

iv) Drug interactions. If you are offered any treatment by another doctor they should be told that you are on AZT.

DDI

DDi is on trial but is likely to receive a product license in the very near future. At present it is available and used in patients who have had to stop AZT usually because of anaemia. It seems DDi may be as effective as AZT.

At present DDi is taken as a powder dissolved in water - with a two hour fast before and thirty minute fast after, as the drug is very sensitive to stomach acid. A sublingual (under the tongue) or a tablet version should be available shortly.

SIDE-EFFECTS

i)   Diarrhoea - severe and uncontrollable diarrhoea through to mild loosening of the bowels. This makes the drug intolerable to some people. It is likely to ease with time and may be due to the antacid used in the preparation rather than the drug itself.

ii) Pancreatitis - inflammation of the pancreas with severe abdominal pain and vomiting. Pancreatitis usually needs a hospital admission. It is more likely in people with quite advanced disease. Pancreatitis may result from HIV rather than the drug.

iii) Peripheral neuropathy - DDi can affect the nerves at the extremities of the body - principally the feet. The commonest symptom is pain. This tends to reverse when the drug is stopped.

iv) Other - it is likely that a similar list of so-called minor side-effects to AZT will be described in time.

It is important to note that the above points i), ii) and iii) may need withdrawal of the drug though it seems often possible to re- start DDi at a lower dose.

DDC

DDc has been on trial in the USA and trials of this used with AZT are starting in UK. DDc seems similar to DDi both in its action and its side-effects. By using it in combination with DDi and AZT low doses of the drugs may be used, so lowering the prevalence of side-effects.

OTHER ANTI-VIRALS - COMBINATION THERAPY

There are a number of other anti-virals being developed. Use of existing drugs is limited by their toxicity in some people and the resistance of some strains of the virus. The future may be the use of a number of different anti-virals in any one person (combination therapy) each at a low dose so reducing side-effects. The management of HIV infection would be similar to diabetes or asthma - the condition cannot be cured, but it can be adequately controlled.

TREATMENT OF OPPORTUNISTIC INFECTIONS AND MALIGNANCIES

1 Pneumocystis carinii pneumonia (PCP)
   PCP is usually treated in hospital with initially intravenous drugs though people with mild infections are increasingly being treated at home.
i) The drug of choice is the antibiotic Septrin (Co-trimoxazole). This can cause nausea, vomiting, gut inflammation, rashes and problems with the blood. It is used at high doses in PCP as it is a life-threatening infection. Septrin is contra-indicated in pregnancy. Septrin can be given by infusion into the veins or by mouth as tablets or suspension. Septrin is usually taken as tablets on alternate days.

ii) Pentamidine is used either by inhalation as a mist or by infusion. It is used in treatment if Septrin cannot be or if the infection does not respond. When used by infusion it can cause serious falls in blood pressure, low blood sugar, blood count problems as well as nausea, vomiting, rashes and so forth. These effects are much less with inhalation as much less of the drug reaches the body. Pentamidine is inhaled from a nebuliser every two weeks. Though the first few doses are taken in a hospital or clinic most people have the equipment necessary at home.

iii) Dapsone is an oral anti-biotic used in combination with trimethoprim. (Trimethoprim is one of the two ingredients in Septrin). Dapsone can cause a peripheral neuropathy (see DDi), skin rashes, loss of appetite, anaemia, headache, insomnia and liver inflammation. Dapsone is taken daily as a tablet.

All three are used to prevent PCP. Anybody at risk is recommended to take one of these - that is people with CD4 cell counts below 200 or people who have had an AIDS-defining illness.

2 CANDIDIASIS (THRUSH)

Thrush is a common fungal infection in HIV disease usually infecting the mouth or vagina. In advanced HIV disease candida can infect most body organs, including the brain. Barrier contraception will protect against re-infection of the vagina.

A number of anti-fungal drugs are available:

i) Amphotericin (Fungilin) is held in the mouth as a lozenge and is effective with mild problems. It is not absorbed from the gut and so does not enter the body. In serious candidiasis it can be used intravenously and is very toxic. It may also cause headaches and generalized muscle aches and pains.

ii) Ketoconazole (Nizoral) are tablets for more serious or difficult to control candidiasis. This may cause nausea, vomiting, abdominal pain, headache, rashes and itching. It may rarely cause very serious liver problems and should not be used in those with liver disease.

iii) Fluconazole (Diflucan) is taken as capsules or an infusion. Can cause nausea, abdominal pain and flatulence. Liver problems have been rarely reported with this drug.

As there is a lack of data these drugs are not recommended in pregnancy or breast-feeding.

3 HERPES INFECTIONS

Herpes infections of the skin and mucous membranes (mouth, vagina and rectum) are common. There is some evidence that repeated infections are detrimental to the immune system, though this is by no means certain. Rarer and more serious infection may occur in body organs particularly the brain.

i) Acyclovir (Zovirax) is effective against the virus but does not eradicate it. It may be used either to treat an infection, or taken continuously to prevent infection. It is available as a tablet or a cream. It is also used intravenously for serious infections.

Side-effects are very unusual. They can be gastro-intestinal disturbance, rises in blood tests measuring liver and kidney function, and fatigue.

Again there is little information on the problems of acyclovir in pregnancy and breast-feeding. Acyclovir can be found in breast milk.

4 CYTOMEGALOVIRUS INFECTION

This is a serious and reasonably common development in advanced HIV disease potentially affecting the eye, bowel and brain. Initially treatment needs to be in hospital with intravenous drugs, continuing at home long-term.

i) Ganciclovir (Cymevene) is used intravenously; can control but not eradicate the infection. People need permanent lines so they can infuse the drug into a vein every or some days.

Ganciclovir causes bone marrow suppression and should not be used with AZT. It is cautioned in use with Septrin. It can also cause facial swelling, nose bleeds, malaise and multiple other side-effects.

ii) Foscarnet sodium (Foscavir) is another intravenous and quite toxic drug. It is used in people who cannot tolerate gangciclovir. Foscarnet should not be used with pentamidine - the combination can cause serious kidney problems.

iv) Prophylaxis. There is no agent available at the moment. An oral version of ganciclovir should be available - its efficiency will then need to be established.

5 CRYPTOSPORIDIUM

A bowel infection causing severe and potentially life-threatening diarrhoea. This organism can found in the tapwater in some areas and particularly in hot periods. Avoidance is advised. Safest is boiling all drinking water (remembering ice, water that fruit or salads are washed in, water in swimming pools). Bottled waters are probably safe and more practical - discuss this with your clinic. Nearly 100 treatments have been tried for Cryptosporidium - none have been effective.

6 CRYPTOCOCCUS

A fungal brain infection. Treatment is by fluconazole (see Candidiasis) or by flucytosine (Alcoban) with amphotericin. This second combination is given initially intravenously, then long-term as tablets to protect against repeated infection. It may cause nausea, vomiting, diarrhoea and rarely bone marrow problems. Though there are benefits in using fluconazole - which is given by mouth rather than by vein - these are probably outweighed by the lower effectiveness of this approach.

7 TOXOPLASMOSIS

Infection by toxoplasma gondii is treated by a combination of an antibiotic and pyrimethamine (Fansidar). Fansidar is then continued as a tablet long term at a lower dose to prevent further infection. It can cause anaemia, skin rashes and insomnia. Treatment of toxoplasma in pregnancy is difficult.

8 LYMPHOMAS

These are a group of malignant diseases of the lymph nodes. They require complex and specialist treatment which cannot be covered here. A combination of treatment by drugs (cytotoxic chemotherapy) and by radiation (radiotherapy) will be advised. These are toxic treatments. General problems are damage to the area of administration, nausea and vomiting, bone marrow suppression, hair loss, fetal deformities if used in pregnancy and rises in uric acid in the blood with a potential for kidney problems.

SUMMARY

While by no means a definitive list of drugs the above are among the most commonly used. When drug treatment is advised ask questions and try to get information from a number of sources. If you have problems with a drug consider lowering the dose. I have not discussed the role of complementary or non-medical interventions. Regular sleep, good diet, stress reduction, moderate exercise and a reduction in smoking and use of other recreational drugs all have benefits. The effects of high dose vitamins, psychotherapy and other healing systems (for example acupuncture, homeopathy) are more controversial, but some people report considerable benefits.

Anyone infected by HIV needs to make their own decisions about their health and interventions to their bodies.

HEALTHY LIVING

KATE THOMSON

*Kate is one of the editors of this book.
She works at Positively Women
and lives in London.*

NO ONE KNOWS why some of us with HIV start getting sick
while others who have been infected for the same length of time
seem to remain healthy. While a healthy lifestyle won't
necessarily prevent illness, it does, none the less, make sense
to do what we can to work at staying fit. But what is a healthy
lifestyle? Sure, we're all told about the importance of taking
care of ourselves when we're diagnosed but what does this mean
in reality? There is no one, simple, easy answer. In fact, the
answer is different for each individual person living with HIV.
It is not a question of rigidly sticking to a list of 'do's' and
'don'ts', but requires working at a delicate and constantly changing balance of needs, desires, and constraints - both mental and
physical. What will seem logical and straightforward for one
person may be unthinkable to the next. There is no right or
wrong - just what is best for you, and what is possible given
your personal situation. What may be practical and affordable
for someone living in a three-bedroomed cottage in Hampstead
may seem like an impossible dream for someone sleeping rough
in Kings Cross. You'll notice that most of the advice here could
apply to anyone, HIV positive or not, trying to stay healthy.

STARTING WITH THE BASICS
There is no way you can reasonably start to take care of your
physical or psychological needs if you don't have a roof over

your head. Even if you do have somewhere to live, your housing may be far from ideal. People with symptomatic HIV disease (ARC or AIDS), may qualify for priority housing from their local boroughs but for people who are asymptomatic this is not usually the case. However, there are several housing associations, such as Strutton in London, who have recognized the importance of preventative help and who will rehouse someone who has no symptoms. There are also ways and means of getting a result through your local authority, although some are more sympathetic than others. The best thing to do is to get in touch with one of the voluntary HIV organizations (for instance, the Terrence Higgins Trust), who have advisers working specifically on housing. You may be able to sort things out through your hospital social worker or a social worker in your local authority (some have special HIV teams), but this often depends on the luck of the draw - some workers are good, others are completely incompetent or indifferent. Once you've found somewhere to live, it's worth checking out the various grants which are available to help furnish your home and also the possibility of getting your local council to pay for telephone installation - again, ask for advice at one of the HIV organizations or see a social worker. If, on the other hand, you do have somewhere suitable to live but because of loss of earnings or other financial problems are having difficulties paying the rent or keeping up mortgage instalments, then it's also important that you seek advice. More often than not, there is a solution and having it worked out will alleviate the stress and worry it's bound to be causing you.

Many people with HIV are struggling to survive on incredibly low incomes. Benefits will never be enough to match someone's needs, but often people are not aware of everything they could be claiming. As with housing, speak to someone who knows what they are talking about, so you are aware of all the options and can apply for what you are entitled to.

DOCTORS AND MEDICAL SERVICES

Being happy with both your hospital and the doctor you see there is vital in terms of optimizing both your physical and mental well-being. Don't be afraid to ask questions, or, if necessary, to change to someone or somewhere else. The more your doctor is willing to explain to you about your condition, the more you will be able to make informed decisions about what you want and the more you will feel in control of things. If you are a drug user or even an ex-user, it's quite likely you will encounter a great deal of hostility and mistrust from medical services. You may be used to this by now, but there is no reason that you should have to put up with discriminatory attitudes - you have the right to expect and receive the same respect and standard of care as anyone else. After all, most of us use drugs of one description or another - alcohol, caffeine, cigarettes. Some drugs are just more socially acceptable than others.

If you do have problems with a particular individual or service you can always go elsewhere. If, however, you don't see why you should have to move when someone else is in the wrong, then think about filing a complaint. After all, if ignorant people are always allowed to get away with it and are never questioned, then they will never change. If you are using street drugs, it's well worth thinking about trying to get scripted instead, as pharmaceuticals are likely to do you far less harm than street gear which is cut with heaven-knows what. If you're injecting, then try to keep a good supply of clean works, as sharing can expose you to a hundred and one other infections. If you do share, then make sure you clean them well with bleach each time they are used, remember to rinse well. Most HIV organizations will be able to point you in the direction of your nearest Drug Dependency Unit (DDU) or needle exchange, but remember - some services will always be more user-friendly than others, so shop around if you can. There is an organization called Mainliners providing services specifically for drug users affected by HIV so it's probably worth getting in touch with them for up-to-date information. They also produce one of the best newsletters around, which they will send you free of charge.

If English is not your first language, then you may experience difficulties communicating with, and understanding your doctor or other staff at your hospital or clinic. If you find that people don't take the time to explain things to you, don't feel bad about asking them to repeat what they're saying as it's important that you know what's going on and why decisions are being made regarding your health. If decisions are consistently made without consulting you or taking into account your wishes and feelings, then something is wrong and you should think about seeing someone else.

Apart from sorting out these basics, what else can you do? Often there is a contradiction between what our body is telling us it needs, and what our head is saying. You may feel tired and know you really should stay home and sleep but psychologically it might feel better to go out and see friends rather than stay on your own. Similarly, you may know that alcohol is no good for the immune system, but still enjoy getting drunk once in a while. The secret is to do as many of the things which are good for your body as often as possible and to do those things which are harmful as infrequently as possible, but without denying yourself everything you enjoy, or forcing yourself to do things you hate. Otherwise you'll be miserable and bored and constantly reminded of the reason why you're making yourself do or not do things - the virus! And if you're feeling like this then your immune system is definitely not being supported one little bit! As you'll probably get sick of hearing again and again - it's all about finding that balance.

Here is a list of things you should be aiming towards. They are usually seen as being 'good' for you. Obviously things which are their opposites are in most circumstances seen as 'bad'. But remember - too much of a good thing can be bad, and a little badness can be good!

THE 'GOOD' LIST
* A healthy diet
  * Adequate sleep and rest
  * Exercise
  * Reducing stress levels
  * Having fun, including safer sex
  * Getting emotional support
  * Getting practical support
  * Complementary therapies
  * Cutting down on tobacco, alcohol and other drugs

A HEALTHY DIET

There's a lot of controversy over this one. No one seems to be able to agree on what is best to eat and what should be avoided. However here are some basic commonsense recommendations which few people would argue with: try to eat as much fresh fruit and vegetables as you can manage without starting to feel like a rabbit. If you cook them, then steam rather than boil them, as this will help to preserve the essential minerals and vitamins. If you have diarrhoea or other problems with your bowels, ease up on these for the moment. You also need to ensure you are getting an adequate intake of protein, so make sure you include this regularly in your diet. Plenty of carbohydrates such as brown rice, wholemeal bread, potatoes, pasta, and pulses, should form a significant part of your diet too. Try out herbal teas, there are so many varieties now that you should be able to find some you like.

Don't aim for a diet which is devoid of anything which gives you eating pleasure. Experiment with herbs and spices. Cut down on sugar but give yourself treats from time to time. Remember that salads don't have to be made up only of boring lettuce leaves, cucumbers and tomatoes. A bit of rice or pasta can be thrown in, some steamed vegetables, different seeds, and unusual bits and pieces of raw vegetables. Yogurt can make a good dressing if you add a little tamari, garlic, and if you're a chilli freak, a dash of something hot. Go for a healthy food basis and then experiment to make it something you really want to eat.

EXERCISE

Exercise is good for all of us. It's most important to find a form you really enjoy. If you don't have much energy then try something gentle, like yoga or non-competitive swimming. It's amazing how afterwards it often leaves you with more energy than you started off with. Check out what's on offer locally, and you'll more than likely find something to suit your taste. And don't forget that going out dancing and having sex are good for exercise too!

REDUCING STRESS LEVELS

Stress is a killer whether you are positive or not, so do what you can to minimize it. Try making a list of the major causes of it in your life and see if you can't take some steps to change these situations (or people), or even avoid them altogether.

Some things we use to help stress, like alcohol or drugs, can be helpful in the short-term but often end up adding to it in the long-term, so watch out! Some tried and tested methods, and voted successful by people we know, include yoga, t'ai c'hi, meditation, hot baths (especially with essential oils added), massage, letting go of anger rather than bottling it up (try smashing something that's not too valuable or having a good scream when the neighbours are out), not letting yourself be talked into doing things you don't want to do (BE ASSERTIVE), visualization and exercise (work out all that aggression in the gym or on the bed!). Do what you can but remember: a stress-free life is an impossibility and anyway a life with no stress at all would probably be a very boring one.

HAVING FUN

Keep busy. Don't tire yourself out by never stopping, day in and day out, but try to ensure your life is full and you have plenty to keep you occupied. Do things you like and that give you a sense of satisfaction and achievement. Do something you've 'always meant to do, but never found the time for'. Find the time. ENJOY YOURSELF.

GETTING EMOTIONAL SUPPORT
Everyone needs someone to talk to about their problems, fears and worries. Sitting and agonizing alone can often lead to feelings getting blown out of proportion. In turn this makes the situation worse. Some people find talking to their health advisers is enough. Others can rely on friends or family. Others go to support groups or for one-to-one counselling for support. However you get it make sure that you do. If you are worried about your children, whether it's a fear for their future, or how and when to tell them about your HIV status, then you may want to get advice and support. There are groups which can offer that. Many of the women who go to Positively Women are mothers and they can share their feelings about their children. Groups which can offer help are listed in the following resource section.

GETTING PRACTICAL SUPPORT
There are loads of different forms of practical support which you may be entitled to. These could range from home-helps, buddies, help with child-minding, shopping and travel. If you have children, you may need specific child care support. You may also want to talk to someone about what plans you have for your children if you get ill. At the back of this book there is a resource list which will enable you to make contact with many of the appropriate organizations which could help you find support. Use it and remember, don't feel guilty about asking for support. The services are there for you to use.

COMPLEMENTARY THERAPIES
Some swear by these. Others are more sceptical. I believe they are often a valuable contribution to well-being. One of the main

drawbacks for many people is the cost involved. However, many AIDS organizations now offer them free of charge, so try them out if you want. Part of the attraction of these therapies is their underlying philosophy. They take a holistic approach towards the individual, treating mind and body as interconnected. Practitioners may advise adopting a special diet and perhaps vitamin supplements or herbal preparations, depending on your medical history and on how you are feeling at the moment. You will find some information on how to find out about complementary therapies in the following resource section.

Many of the chapters in this book include experiences, information and advice which women living with HIV and AIDS may find useful. Be kind to yourself and get as much support as you need and want. Good luck!

RESOURCES
&
READING LIST

Compiled by Hope Massiah,
with help from Chris Arnephie,
Pat Adams and Becky Shaw.

The information in this section is compiled in the following order:

All information is listed alphabetically within each section.

SUPPORT AND COUNSELLING SERVICES

AIDS AHEAD
144 London Road
Northwich
CHESHIRE CW9 5HH
0606-47047
0606-330472 (minicom)
LONDON 081-348 9195
081-342 8791(minicom)
Counselling and support
services for deaf people.

**AIDS HELPLINE
NORTHERN IRELAND**
0232 326117
Minicom available, also face-
to-face counselling.

**BLACK HIV/AIDS
NETWORK (BHAN)**
111 Devonport Road
LONDON W12 8PB
081-749 2828
Counselling in Hindi, Urdu,
Bengali, Gujerati and
Swahili. Counselling can be
arranged in Thai,
Vietnamese, Amharic,
Punjabi, Cantonese, Arabic
and Chinese dialects.

BLACKLINERS
PO Box 1274
LONDON SW9 8EX
071-738 5274
Support for African,
Caribbean and Asian people.

BODY POSITIVE
51b Philbeach Gardens
LONDON SW5 9EB
071-835 1045
(or 071-373 9124
7-10 p.m.)
Body Positive
Women's Group:
071-370 2051
Positive Youth:
071-373 7547
Support counselling and
advice for people who are
HIV positive, also has details
of Body Positive groups and
services nationwide.

THE FOOD CHAIN
071-250 1391
London-wide organization
providing hot meals to
housebound people with
HIV/AIDS and their carers.
Currently Sundays only.
Referrals can be made
through other HIV/AIDS
organizations and the Social
Services HIV team.

**GOFAL SDIC GOGLEDD
CYMRU (AIDS CARE
NORTH WALES)**
PO Box 470
Llandudno
GWYNEDD
LL30 1RL
0492-860569
Helpline

GRANDMA'S
P O Box 1392
LONDON SW6 4EJ
A service for children
affected by HIV and AIDS.

HAEMOPHILIA SOCIETY
123 Westminster
Bridge Road
LONDON SE1 7HR
071-928 2020
Information, advice and
support for everyone who has
haemophilia - and special
representation of people
infected with HIV through
using Factor 8.

THE LANDMARK
47 Tulse Hill
LONDON SW2
081-671 7611
Day centre for people who
have HIV infection and
people who have AIDS.
Offer meals and recreational
facilities. Women only
evening.

LONDON LIGHTHOUSE
111 - 117 Lancaster Road
LONDON W11 1QT
071-792 1200
A centre for all people facing
the challenge of AIDS.
Counselling, support groups,
drop-in facility, play group,
residential care, training.

MAINLINERS
PO Box 125
LONDON SW9 8EF
071-737 3141
Support for people affected
by HIV and drugs (including
alcohol).

NATIONAL AIDS HELPLINE
(FREE PHONE)
0800-567123 24 hours
0800-521361 minicom
10 a.m. to 10 p.m.
0800-282445
Bengali, Gujerati, Hindi,
Punjabi, Urdu and English
Weds 6-10 p.m.
0800-282446
Cantonese and English
Tues 6-10 p.m.
0800-282447
Arabic and English
Weds 6-10 p.m.

NURSES SUPPORT GROUP
071-708 5605
Mon and Weds 7-10 p.m.
Runs helpline for nursing
staff needing advice and help
with HIV and AIDS
problems.

PACE (PROJECT FOR
ADVICE, COUNSELLING
AND INFORMATION)
c/o LLGC
see OTHER RELATED
ORGANIZATIONS for
address.
071-251 2689
Free counselling for lesbians
and gay men.

POSITIVE OPTIONS
354 Goswell Road
LONDON EC1V 7LQ
071-278 5039
A Barnardos scheme
providing information,
advice and support for
families where one or both
parents are HIV positive and
who need help in making
plans for the future care of
their children. Also work
with children and their
families/guardians where a
child is HIV positive. The
scheme is confidential and
independent. Projects
nationwide. Phone for details.

**POSITIVE PARTNERS AND
POSITIVELY CHILDREN**
The Annexe
Jan Rebane Centre
12-14 Thornton Street
LONDON SW9 0BL
071-738 7333

**POSITIVE WOMEN
SCOTLAND**
EDINBURGH:
c/o SCOTTISH AIDS
MONITOR
64 Broughton Street
EDINBURGH EH1 3SA
031-557 3885

GLASGOW:
c/o SCOTTISH AIDS
MONITOR
22 Woodside Terrace
GLASGOW G3 7XB
041-353 3133
Scottish AIDS Monitor also

provides a full range of
advice, information and
support services.

**POSITIVELY IRISH
ACTION ON AIDS**
St Margaret's House
21 Old Ford Rd
LONDON E2 9PL
081-983 0192 (admin line)
081-983 4293 (referrals)
Support and information for
Irish People affected by HIV/
AIDS in the UK.

POSITIVELY WOMEN
5 Sebastian Street
LONDON EC1V OHE
071 490 5501 (Admin)
071 490 5515 (Client
Services)
071 490 2327 (Helpline:
Mondays to Fridays
12-2 p.m.)
Positively Women provides a
range of support and
counselling services to
women who are HIV positive
and to children directly
affected by HIV.

Services provided:
* Individual counselling and
support to women who are
HIV positive including
prison and hospital visits.
* Support Groups. For further
details see below.
* Childrens Fund, small grants
for the benefit of children
affected by HIV/AIDS.
* Housing advice and referrals
* Welfare rights advice

* Alternative therapies
* Leaflets on women's HIV
  issues. To date these are:
  AFRICAN WOMENS
  HEALTH ISSUES;
  PREVENTION; A
  POSITIVE RESULT?;
  WOMEN DRUGS AND
  HIV; PREGNANCY AND
  CHILDCARE.
* Children's worker, support to
  children affected by HIV
  (Part of Barnardos' Positive
  Options team).
* Speakers Bureau
* Training on Women and HIV
  issues

SUPPORT GROUPS - Please
phone the office for details.
WEEKLY
Monday: 2 - 4 p.m.
Venue: Hammersmith,
WEST LONDON
Wednesday: 6.30 - 8 p.m.
Venue: The Landmark,
SOUTH LONDON
Thursday: 6.30 - 8.30 p.m.
Venue: Positively Women,
NORTH LONDON
FORTNIGHTLY
African Women's Support
Group 2nd and 4th Friday of
every month
Time: 11 a.m. - 1 p.m.
Venue: Positively Women,
NORTH LONDON
MONTHLY
East London Women's
Support Group 1st Friday of
the month
Time: 6-9 p.m.
Venue: Mansfield Settlement,

EAST LONDON
OPEN AFTERNOONS
For clients and their friends
Thursdays bi-weekly
Time: 12-5 p.m.
Venue: Positively Women,
NORTH LONDON
Lunch and massage provided

THE WOMEN'S GROUP
PO Box 201
MANCHESTER M60 1PU
061-839 4340
Support group for HIV
positive women in the North
West of England.

**SHARE (SHAKTI HIV/AIDS
RESPONSE)**
c/o The Landmark
See above for address.
081-678 6686
A support group for South
Asian people with HIV.

SHEPERDESS WALK
100 Shepherdess Walk
LONDON N1 7JN
071-250 1390
A community based service
for people affected by HIV/
AIDS. The voluntary
organizations based here are:
BLACKLINERS, POSITIVE
PARTNERS, POSITIVELY
CHILDREN and THE FOOD
CHAIN.

TERRENCE HIGGINS TRUST
52-54 Grays Inn Road
LONDON WC1 8JU
071-831 0330
071-242 1010 (helpline)
071-405 2381
(legal line: 7-10 p.m.
Wednesdays) 0800-212529
(prisoners link: 3-6 p.m.
Tuesdays and Thursdays)
Practical support, help, counselling and advice for people with or people concerned about HIV and AIDS.

Your local HIV organization, genito-urinary medical clinic, doctor, social services etc. should be able to put you in touch with counselling and support services in your area.

HOLISTIC/COMPLEMENTARY THERAPIES

These are wide range of therapies which, with a few exceptions, are dismissed by the Western medical establishment. Many have been used for thousands of years and they are often used by people with HIV and AIDS.
They tend to focus on the whole person rather than symptoms and unlike conventional treatments for HIV/AIDS they rarely have nasty side -effects.
Unfortunately few of them are available on the National Health and so might be difficult to afford.
It is important to make sure that the therapist you choose is properly trained.
Your local HIV/AIDS organization or centre may be able to give you information about therapies that people with HIV/AIDS have found helpful and suggest therapists. They may also provide complementary therapies free or at low cost. If you are going to use complementary therapies seek advice and let your NHS doctor know what you are doing.

SOME TYPES OF THERAPY

ACUPUNCTURE
A technique of traditional Chinese medicine, using very fine needles which are inserted into the body. This stimulates points on the bodies surface which has a beneficial effect on the bodies functioning.

AUTOGENIC TRAINING
A system of attention focusing exercises designed to generate a state of mind and body relaxation.

COLONIC IRRIGATION/COLON HYDROTHERAPY
Water enters the colon via a tube inserted into the anus (bum) under gentle pressure. Helps to cleanse the body of poison producing waste materials.

HERBAL REMEDIES
The use of plants in various forms, dried, teas, oils, tinctures, etc, for the relief of certain ailments or to improve general health. For example, goldenseal and liquorice are thought to strengthen the immune system.

HOMEOPATHY
Based on the principle 'like cures like', substances that cause certain symptoms in a healthy person are given to someone suffering from similar symptoms. Homeopathic remedies are extremely diluted and are made from plants, animal materials and natural chemicals.

MASSAGE
Therapeutic stroking and kneading of the body usually using oils. There are many different forms including Swedish, shiatsu and aromatherapy, where essential aromatic oils are used. Good for stress, muscular tension and general well-being.

NATUROPATHY
A branch of alternative medicine that encourages the body's own ability to heal itself by using diet, relaxation, breathing excercises, herbs, or other treatments appropriate to the individual patient.

NUTRITION THERAPIES
Using diet and nutritional supplements (e.g. vitamins) as tools in preventative and therapeutic medicine.

HEALTH FOUNDATIONS

COMMUNITY HEALTH FOUNDATION
The East West Centre
188 Old Street
LONDON EC1V 9BP
071-251 4076
A charity offering various complementary therapies at reasonable prices.

IMMUNE DEVELOPMENT TRUST
The Basement
Gatestone
Cromer Street
LONDON WC1H 8EA
071-837 2151
A registered charity which provides holistic therapies for people with AIDS, HIV, cancer and other immune-related illnesses.

NORTHERN LIGHTS TRUST
BM Breathe
LONDON WC1N 3XX
0992-576649
AIDS mastery workshops
which focus on visualization
and other healing techniques.

SOLAS
2/4 Abbeymount
EDINBURGH EH8 8EJ
031-661 0982
An HIV centre with a full
range of services including
complementary therapies.

The following can provide information on local practitioners:

**BRITISH ACUPUNCTURE
ASSOCIATION**
34 Alderney Street
LONDON SW1V 4EU
071-834 1012
071-834 6229

**BRITISH HOMEOPATHIC
ASSOCIATION**
27a Devonshire Street
LONDON W1 1RJ
071-935 2163
Has lists of GPs, dentists and
pharmacists who practise
homeopathy and NHS
hospitals where homeopathy
is available.

**INSTITUTE FOR
COMPLEMENTARY
MEDICINE**
PO Box 194
LONDON SE16 1QZ
071-237 5165

Has a register of practitioners
of many complementary
therapies.

**NATIONAL FEDERATION
OF SPIRITUAL HEALERS**
Old Manor Farm Studio
Church Street
Sunbury on Thames
MIDDLESEX TW16 6RG
0932-783164
Spiritual healing provided
free to people who are HIV
positive. Donations
welcome.

CAROL SMITH
11 Painsthorpe Road
LONDON N16
071-254 4248
A practising naturopath and
osteopath. Appointments
only.

SAFER SEX: CONDOMS, DENTAL DAMS

Free condoms are available from:

Local HIV Services and self help groups such as your local
Body Positive Group.

Family Planning Clinics, look them up in the phone book.

Brook Advisory Centres

Needle Exchanges

Genito-Urinary (STD) Clinics

Well Woman Clinics

DENTAL DAMS/ORAL SHIELDS:
This a 15 cm square of latex which makes oral sex or rimming (mouth to anus sex) safer. You place it over a woman's vulva or woman's anus. They are called dental dams because they are used by dentists to place in a patient's mouth.

Free dental dams are not so readily available but you may be able to get dental dams free from local HIV services.

POSITIVELY WOMEN
(See SUPPORT AND COUNSELLLING SERV-ICES above) *will supply free condoms and dental dams to HIV positive women.*

You can buy/order dental dams from:

COLLONNADES CHEMISTS
28 Porchester Rd
LONDON W2 6ES
071-727 5713

CONDOMANIA
Condoms, dental dams, gloves etc are all available at CONDOMANIA shops in LEEDS, LIVERPOOL and LONDON.

LEEDS
The Balcony
The Corn Exchange
Call Lane
LEEDS LS1
0532-446532

LIVERPOOL
Liverpool Palace
6-10 Slater Street
LIVERPOOL L1
051-707 0189

LONDON
57 Rupert Street
LONDON W1
071-287 4540

HEALTH CO. UK LTD.
196 Great Cambridge Rd
ENFIELD
Middlesex EN1 1UN
081-366 4412

Safer sex information and
leaflets are obtainable from:

**TERRENCE HIGGINS
TRUST**
(See SUPPORT AND
COUNSELLING
SERVICES above)

WOMEN'S HEALTH
(See RELATED
ORGANIZATIONS below)

**LESBIAN AND GAY
SWITCHBOARD**
(See RELATED
ORGANIZATIONS below)

INFORMATION FOR EX AND CURRENT DRUG USERS

ANGEL PROJECT
38-44 Liverpool Road
LONDON N1 0PU
071-226 3113
Advice and information for
people with drug related
problems. Syringe exchange.
Free dental dams and
condoms. Women only
sessions.

BIRMINGHAM DRUGS LINE
Dale House
New Meeting Street
BIRMINGHAM B4 7SX
021-632 6363

BRIDGE PROJECT
154 Mill Road
CAMBRIDGE CB1 3LP
0223-214614

BRISTOL DRUGS PROJECT
18 Guinea Street
Redcliffe
BRISTOL BS1 6SX
0272-298047
0272-298048 (Admin)

**DUNAIN HOUSE
ADDICTION UNIT**
Craig Dunain Hospital
INVERNESS
Scotland IV3
0463-234101 x2218

EXETER DRUGS PROJECT
The 59 Centre
59 Magdalen Street
EXETER EX2 4HY
0392-410292

**LIVERPOOL
SYRINGE EXCHANGE**
Merseyside Regional AIDS
Prevention
Maryland Centre
8 Maryland Street
LIVERPOOL L1 9BX
051-709 2231

MAINLINERS
See SUPPORT & COUN-
SELLING SEVICES above
Support and information for
people affected by HIV and
drugs (including alcohol).

NARCOTICS ANONYMOUS
PO Box 417
LONDON SW10 0RS
071-351 6794 (Helpline)

**NORTH EAST COUNCIL
FOR ADDICTIONS/WOMEN
AND ALCOHOL**
1 Mosley Street
NEWCASTLE
-UPON-TYNE
091-232 7878 (Counselling)
091-232 0797 (Information)

SCODA
Standing Conference on
Drug Abuse
1 - 4 Hatton Place
LONDON EC1N 8ND
071-430 2341
HIV information officer with
lists of needle exchange

schemes throughout the
country.

**TIM CYFFURIAU
CYMUNEDOL
COMMUNITY DRUG TEAM/**
Community Drug Clinic
46 Cowbridge Road East
Canton
CARDIFF CF1 9DU
0222-395877/8

**WOMEN AND AIDS
DRUG DEPENDANTS
ANONYMOUS**
Drug Dependents Anony-
mous
1 Newcastle Chambers
Off Angel Row
NOTTINGHAM NG1 3HQ
0602-412888

INFORMATION FOR SEX WORKERS

CENTENARY PROJECT
37 Henderson Hse
Leith
EDINBURGH
031-553 2490
Support and non-judgemental
counselling to women
working in prostitution,
HIV counselling and testing.

**CLASH (CENTRAL LONDON
ACTION ON STREET
HEALTH)**
15 Bateman Buildings
Soho Hospital
Soho Square
LONDON W1V 5TW
071-734 1794
Counselling, medical services
and advice for young people.

MARYLAND CENTRE
8 Maryland St
LIVERPOOL L1 9BX
051-709 2231
Support, information and
health care for women who
work on the streets.

PRAED STREET PROJECT
c/o Jeffries Wing
St Mary's Hospital
LONDON W2 1NY
071-725 1549
Confidential STD checks,
and general women's health
service for sex workers.
Drop-in facility on
Wednesday and Thursday
2-6 p.m.

SAFE:
PROSTITUTE RESEARCH/
OUTREACH PROJECT
South Birmingham Health
Authority
Vincent Drive
Edgbaston
BIRMINGHAM B15 2TZ
021-627 2058
021-359 0653 (Well woman
clinic)
Drop In :
213 Mary Street
Balsall Heath
BIRMINGHAM B12
021-440 4040
Support, information and
advice for women working in
the sex industry.

SCOTTISH PROSTITUTES
EDUCATION PROJECT
(SCOT-PEP)
21a Torphichen Street
EDINBURGH EH3 8HX
031-229 8269
Support, advice and
information for people who
work in the sex industry.

SHEFFIELD AIDS EDUCA-
TION PROJECT
37 Stone Grove
SHEFFIELD
S10 2SW
0742-754038
Drop-in, advice, information
and support for women who
work in the sex industry.

ADVICE AND LEGAL   ISSUES

IMMUNITY
260a Kilburn Lane
LONDON W10 4BA
081-968 8909
Free legal and welfare advice
from lawyers on any problem
associated with HIV/AIDS.

REFUGEE COUNCIL
3 Bond Way
LONDON SW8 1SJ
071-582 6922
071-582 1162 (Refugee
helpline 2-5 p.m.)
071-582 9927 (Refugee advisors support unit 10 a.m.
to 1 p.m.)

RELEASE
388 Old Street
LONDON EC1V 9LT
071-729 9904 (office hours)
071-603 8654 (evenings and
weekends)
Advice and information on
drug related problems.

SCOTTISH AIDS MONITOR
64 Broughton Street
EDINBURGH EH1 3SA
031-557 3885
Advisory legal bureau on
AIDS.

SUSSEX AIDS CENTRE
Graham Wilkerson House
PO Box 17
BRIGHTON
East Sussex BN2 5NQ
0273-608511
Legal and welfare rights
advice.

**TERRENCE HIGGINS
TRUST**
For details see SUPPORT
AND COUNSELLING
SERVICES above,
Advice and practical help on
any legal problem to do with
HIV/AIDS.

**UK IMMIGRANTS
ADVISORY SERVICE**
2nd Floor
County House
Great Dover Street
LONDON SE1 4YB
071-357 6917
081-759 9234 (Emergency
outside office hours)
Provides HIV/AIDS advice
and information for
immigrants to the UK.

You may also get advice from your local HIV organization, Citizens Advice Bureau or Law Centre, with non-HIV organizations you will need to think about whether you want to disclose your HIV status.

BENEFITS AND GRANTS

Many people who are HIV positive are well and may be working, but for some people who are occasionally sick or who may be unable to carry on with full-time employment it is important to get advice to be sure you are claiming all the benefits that you are entitled to.

Benefits that people with HIV/AIDS may be entitled to:

Attendance Allowance - for people who need help with things like getting dressed, eating, going to the toilet, etc.

Child Benefit - for people who have responsibility for children under sixteen or under nineteen and still in full-time education.

Community Charge (Poll Tax) rebate - for people on low incomes, employed or not.

Family Credit - for people on low incomes who have responsibility for children.

Housing Benefit - for people on low incomes, employed or not.

Income Support - for people on low incomes, employed or not.

Invalid Care Allowance - for people who are spending at least thirty-five hours a week caring for someone on Attendance Allowance.

Invalidity Benefit - for people on long-term sick leave from work or unemployed people who have signed off sick for six months.

Mobility Allowance - for people who have difficulty walking or are unable to walk.

One Parent Benefit - for people with sole responsibility for children.

Severe Disablement Allowance - unless you are blind, partially sighted or profoundly deaf you have to have a medical assessment for this benefit.

Sickness Benefit - for people who are unemployed and unwell.

Social Fund - community care grants, crisis loans, funeral payments.

Statutory Sick Pay - for people who are employed and off work on sick leave.

Travel - taxi cards and travel passes

Unemployment Benefit - for people who are unemployed and have paid enough National Insurance contributions to qualify.

All of the above benefits may not cover the cost of essential items such as electricity bills or childrens clothing. Other problems could be delays in applying for, or receiving payments, and/or a changing state of health. Many HIV organizations such as BODY POSITIVE, POSITIVELY WOMEN and TERRENCE HIGGINS TRUST (See SUPPORT AND COUNSELLING SERVICES above) give grants to people who are HIV positive, to help out with necessities. Check also with your local HIV organization.

HOUSING INFORMATION

Many HIV/AIDS organizations, including POSITIVELY WOMEN have specialist housing workers who can give advice or make referrals for housing.

BLACKLINERS
For details see SUPPORT AND COUNSELLING SERVICES above.
For black people of African and Asian descent.

HOMELESS ACTION
52-54 Featherstone Street
LONDON EC1Y 8RT
071-251 6783
Provides medium-term housing for homeless women.

LLINELL GYMORTH AIDS CAERDYDD
(CARDIFF AIDS HELPLINE)
57 Crwys Road
CARDIFF
0222-223443 Minicom available
0222-666465 evenings 7-10 p.m.
Information and housing referrals.

PICCADILLY ADVICE CENTRE
100 Shaftesbury Avenue
LONDON W1 7DH
071-434 3773 2-6 p.m. and 7-9 p.m. (every day of the year)
Information and referrals to people who are homeless or new to LONDON.

STRUTTON HOUSING ASSOCIATION
8 Strutton Ground
LONDON SW1P 2HP
071-222 5921
A specialist housing association for people who are HIV positive. Please note that there is no waiting list and direct referrals are not accepted.

SUPPORTED ACCOMODATION TEAM AIDS (SATA)
20 Albany Street
EDINBURGH EH1 3QB
031-556 9140
Supportive housing for people with HIV/AIDS.

TERRENCE HIGGINS TRUST (LEGAL SERVICES)
For details see SUPPORT AND COUNSELLING SERVICES above.

THRESHOLD HOUSING ASSOCIATION
467 Garratt Lane
LONDON SW18 4SN
081-874 1680
A general housing agency which provides support and housing to people who are HIV positive.

IMMIGRATION AND TRAVEL

Many countries have some sort of restriction of travel or entry to people who are HIV positive, or thought to be.

If you have reason to believe that you might be HIV positive or you are likely to be thought to HIV positive it may be worth ringing the Embassy or Consulate of the destination country to check the current situation.

**FOREIGN OFFICE
CONSULAR SERVICE**
Clive House
Petty France
LONDON SW1
071-270 4129
071-270 4151
(Weekends, 9-5 p.m.)
071-270 3000
(Emergency number
for out of office hours)
Information for British
Citizens about travel
restrictions, immunizations,
health and safety issues etc.

**JOINT COUNCIL
FOR THE WELFARE
OF IMMIGRANTS (JCWI)**
115 Old Street
LONDON EC1V 9JR
071-251 8706
(Weekdays 2-5 p.m.,
except Wednesday).
Information and advice on all
matters related to
immigration in UK.

NATIONAL RESTRICTIONS

This is a list of some of the countries that have restrictions.

AUSTRALIA
HIV positive people who apply for permanent residency are assessed on economic and other grounds.

CANADA
A few HIV positive people have been refused entry, but officially they don't have routine tests for HIV.

CHINA
Long-term foreign residents are tested on arrival.

CYPRUS
African students and people entering to work in nightclubs are tested on arrival.

INDIA
Foreign students and long-term visitors are tested on arrival.

NIGERIA
HIV positive citizens of any country that requires testing of Nigerian citizens will be refused entry.

PAKISTAN
Long-term foreign visitors are tested.

TURKEY
People known to have HIV are refused entry.

UK
'Visitors suspected of having HIV' have been refused entry. Potential immigrants can be required by an immigration officer to submit to a medical examination. If found to be HIV positive they are likely to be excluded on the grounds that they may be unable to pay for medical treatment they may require. (For immigration advice services see also ADVICE AND BENEFITS.

USA
Applicants for residency are tested. People known to have HIV are refused residency and tourist visas (with a few exceptions).

OTHER RELATED ORGANIZATIONS

ACT-UP (AIDS Coalition to Unleash Power)
c/o LLGC - see below for address
071-490 5749
A direct action group which meets every Tuesday evening at the LLGC.

address
071-490 7153
A direct action group for the rights of lesbians and gay men which meets every Thursday evening at the LLGC.

LONDON LESBIAN AND GAY CENTRE (LLGC)
67-69 Cowcross Road
LONDON EC1
071-608 1471

LONDON LESBIAN AND GAY SWITCHBOARD
BM Switchboard
LONDON WC1N 3XX
071-837 7324
OUTRAGE
c/o LLGC - see above for

RAPE CRISIS CENTRE
P O Box 69
LONDON WC1
071-837 1600 (24 hours)
Physical protection and emotional support.

THE UK COALITION
OF PEOPLE LIVING
WITH HIV/AIDS
   c/o LONDON LIGHT-
   HOUSE - See SUPPORT
   AND COUNSELLING
   SERVICES for address
   071-792 1200

WOMEN'S HEALTH
(formerly WHRRIC)
   52-54 Featherstone Street
   LONDON EC1Y 8RT
   071-251 6580
   A library of information on
   womens health issues
   including HIV.

SOURCES OF INFORMATION ABOUT TREATMENT AND OTHER HIV/AIDS ISSUES

FREE INFORMATION:

AVERT
   AIDS Education and
   Research Trust
   P O Box 91
   Horsham
   WEST SUSSEX RH13 7YR
   0403-864010

BLACK HIV/AIDS
NETWORK NEWSLETTER
   111 Devonport Road
   Shepherds Bush
   LONDON W12 8PB
   071-749 2828

BODY POSITIVE
NEWS-LETTER
   51b Philbeach Gardens
   LONDON SW5 9EB
   071-835 1045

MAINLINERS NEWS-
LETTER
   PO Box 125
   LONDON SW9 8EF
   071-737 3141
   Free to positive people and
   drug users.

PINK PAPER
   77 City Garden Row
   LONDON N1
   071-608 2566
   Available free in many
   lesbian and gay meeting
   places.

NOT FREE:

AIDS DIALOGUE
   Health Education
   Authority
   Hamilton House
   Mabledon Place
   LONDON WC1H 9TX
   071-383 3833

AIDS TREATMENT NEWS
   PO Box 411256
   San Francisco
   CA 94141
   USA
   Information on the latest
   treatment.

BRITISH MEDICAL
JOURNAL (BMJ)
  British Medical Association
  Tavistock Square
  LONDON WC1H 9JR
  071-387 4499
  A medical journal.

HIV NEWS REVIEW
  Information Department
  TERRENCE HIGGINS
  TRUST
  For details see SUPPORT
  AND COUNSELLING
  SERVICES above.

THE LANCET
  42 Bedford Square
  LONDON WC1B 3SL
  071-436 4981
  A weekly medical journal.

NATIONAL AIDS MANUAL
  NAM Publications Ltd
  Unit 136
  Brixton Enterprise Centre
  LONDON SW9 8EJ
  071-737 1846
  Three large volumes, though
  the women's section is very
  slim. Expensive for one
  person, but most large HIV
  organizations should have it.

WORLD (WOMEN
ORGANIZING TO
RESPOND TO LIFE
THREATENING DISEASES)
  PO Box 11535
  Oakland
  CA 94611
  USA
  A newsletter for and about
  women facing HIV.

Your local library or HIV organization may keep the above publications
or other up-to-date information about HIV.

FURTHER READING

MAKING IT: A Woman's Guide to Sex in the Age of AIDS
Eds. Cindy Patton and Janis Kelly. Bilingual Spanish/English.
(Crossing Press, USA, 1987, £2.50)

**MATTERS OF LIFE AND DEATH
(WOMEN SPEAK ABOUT AIDS)**
Eds. Ines Reider and Patricia Ruppelt
(Virago, £6.50)

POSITIVE WOMEN: Voices of Women Living With AIDS
(Second Story, Canada)

SAFER SEX: The Guide For Women Today
Diane Richardson (Pandora, £7.99)

WOMEN, AIDS AND ACTIVISM
Eds. ACT-UP/New York Women and AIDS Book Group.
(South End Press, USA, £6.95)

WOMEN AND THE AIDS CRISIS
Diane Richardson (Pandora, £4.95) Revised edition.

WOMEN, RISK AND AIDS PROJECT (WRAP)
A series of pamphlets concentrating on exploring the sexual practices,
beliefs and understanding of young women, especially in relation to HIV
and AIDS.
The WRAP team is: Janet Holland, Caroline Ramazanoglu,
Sue Scott, Sue Sharpe and Rachel Thomson.
The Tufnell Press, 47 Dalmany Road, LONDON N7 0DY.

WORKING WITH WOMEN AND AIDS
(Forthcoming from Routledge, Autumn 1992).

GLOSSARY

This glossary is by no means comprehensive, but is a list of the most common terms or abbreviations used in the book. All information is correct at time of printing.

AIDS

Acquired Immune Deficiency Syndrome. It is a condition in which the immune system is broken down. This can mean that the body's ability to fight disease is lessened, leaving individuals vulnerable to infections and/or cancers which may be life threatening. There is a list of 120 or so specific opportunistic infections or malignancies, one or more of which will result in an official diagnosis of AIDS.

ARC

A loose categorization of AIDS-related symptoms that are linked to HIV infection but are not included in the specific case definition of AIDS by the CDC. The differentiation between people with ARC and people with AIDS is significant because many social services, are dependent of an official AIDS diagnosis, and are not otherwise available to people with ARC, even though they might show serious disabling symptoms. A term in disfavour among AIDS activists, as it is understood to impose distinctions artificially among people with HIV-related illness.

AZT

Azidothymidine, Zidovudine Retrovir. This is, at present, the only licensed anti-HIV anti-viral drug.

DDi

Didanosine (Dideoxy inosine) is an anti-viral drug currently on trial in the UK. It is now licensed in the USA.

GP

Abbreviation of General Practitioner. Otherwise known as the family doctor.

HIV

Human immunodeficiency virus. This is the virus which many experts believe can lead to AIDS. Not everyone who has HIV seems to develop AIDS. HIV may be present in the body for a number of years before signs of illness or infection appear.

PCP

Pneumocystis carinii pneumonia. This is a life-threatening infection common in HIV-related illness. With proper treatment and preventative measures can be controlled, often by prophylaxis.

PROPHYLAXIS

Preventative treatment. This is a general medical term for the use of treatment as prevention, e.g. as aerosolized pentamadine is used for PCP.

REHAB

Common abbreviation for drug rehabilitation unit. A place where people addicted to drugs undergo detoxification under medical and social supervision.

STD

Sexually transmitted disease. This is an umbrella term for any disease that can be contracted through sexual activity, such as gonorrhoea, syphilis, herpes, hepatitis B, etc.

T-CELL

This is a type of white cell in the blood that activates the rest of the immune system. A T-cell count is the principal test in detecting evidence of a decline in immunity. Other names are are T4- cell and/or CD4-cell.

EDITORS'
BIOGRAPHIES

SUE O'SULLIVAN has lived in London for thirty years. Even so, she has never lost her American accent which she attributes to either 'strength of character' or pigheadedness. She has two grown-up sons and lives in short-life housing in Kings Cross. She has edited a number of books, including Sheba's feminist cookbook *Turning the Tables,* and Virago's *Out the Other Side, Contemporary Lesbian Writing,* with Christian McEwan. For five years she was part of the Sheba team, leaving in Autumn 1991 to pursue a busy but financially unsuccessful freelance career. She has been involved in health issues since the 1970s, has a health education diploma, and has worked around HIV and AIDS and women's sexuality since the early 1980s.

KATE THOMSON, aged thirty-one, is a founder member of Positively Women and has been diagnosed since 1987. She now works full-time as Project Manager for Positively Women and also takes an active role in national and international HIV conferences as well as speaking around the world on behalf of women living with HIV. When she is not taking good care of her physical well-being, she has been known to get drunk and behave outrageously. She lives in a flat in north London with a spectacular view of Holloway Prison.

FORTHCOMING AND RECENT TITLES FROM SHEBA

These books are available from most good bookshops or by mail order from SHEBA, 10A BRADBURY STREET, LONDON N16 8JN. Please send cheque or postal order and add 85p p&p per book.

POSITIVELY WOMEN: LIVING WITH AIDS, Eds. O'Sullivan and Thomson
ISBN 0 907179 47 9 £9.99 May 1992

For the first time in the UK, in their own words, a variety of women tell how they coped with the devastating news that they were HIV positive. As well as moving personal testimony and experience the book also includes factual advice on housing, treatment and other issues as well as a comprehensive resource list.

THE GILDA STORIES, Jewelle Gomez
ISBN 0 907179 61 4 £7.99 June 1992

An American odyssey, a romantic adventure, a magical tale that sweeps you along as the immortal Gilda strides across time. A unique vampire, Gilda listens to the world and tries to add her own voice. History offers cataclysms and everyday horrors but it also offers community and kindred spirits.

WILD HEARTS, The Wild Hearts Group
ISBN 0 907179 59 2 6.99 October 1991

The first collection of original melodrama of its kind: passionate, intriguing, witty, bitter-sweet stories to capture the imagination. These wildly imaginative writers have produced a thoroughly engaging volume which speaks to the inexorable rise and fall of the lesbian heartbeat.

GIRLS, VISIONS AND EVERYTHING, Sarah Schulman
ISBN 0 907179 58 4 £6.99 November 1991

This is a sexy and spirited novel from the author of AFTER DELORES, PEOPLE IN TROUBLE and THE SOPHIE HOROWITZ STORY (also published by SHEBA). With her keys in her pocket and a copy of On The Road in her hand, Lila Futuransky is looking for adventure....